PLEASING THE PATIENT

Geoff Watts has been a writer and broadcaster on medical subjects since 1971, and is best known as the presenter of *Medicine Now* on BBC Radio 4. He won Glaxo Science Writing Awards in 1974 and 1984, and has four times won the Medical Journalists Association Radio Award. Geoff Watts lives in Hampstead, London.

PLEASING THE PATIENT

GEOFF WATTS

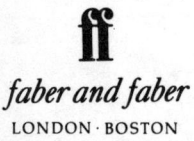

faber and faber
LONDON · BOSTON

First published in 1992
by Faber and Faber Limited
3 Queen Square London WC1N 3AU

Phototypeset by Intype Ltd, London
Printed in England by Clays Ltd, St Ives plc

All rights reserved

© Geoff Watts, 1992

Geoff Watts is hereby identified as author of this work in accordance with Section 77 of the Copyright, Designs and Patents Act 1988

This book is sold subject to the condition that it shall not, by way of trade or otherwise, be lent, resold, hired out or otherwise circulated without the publisher's prior consent in any form of binding or cover other than that in which it is published and without a similar condition including this condition being imposed on the subsequent purchaser.

A CIP record for this book
is available from the British Library

ISBN 0–571–16441–2

Contents

Acknowledgements   vii
Introduction   viii

PART ONE: The Placebo Effect

1 Pink Pills and Friendly Physicians   3
2 A Tiresome Distraction   23
3 The Healing Mind   30

PART TWO: Two Styles of Medicine

4 Into the Consulting Rooms   51
5 A Crooked Path   60
6 A Series of Rebellions   73

PART THREE: One Medicine

7 Who Are the Healers Now?   95
8 Harnessing the Placebo Effect   117
9 Mainstream Meets the Fringe   139
10 To Please the Patient   148

References   165
Index   171

Acknowledgements

My thanks to Lucinda Culpin of June Hall Literary Agency, Roger Osborne of Faber and Faber, and the many practitioners – orthodox and complementary – who agreed to talk to me.

Introduction
A sad divide – and how to overcome it

Consider these paradoxes, most of them everyday events in medicine:

- When pills identical in all respects except their colour are given to two groups of patients, those taking pills of one colour sometimes do consistently better than those taking pills of the other colour.
- When doctors assess the benefits of a new drug by comparing its effects with those of a dummy preparation, some patients who have received only the dummy pill also show an improvement.
- When the Government decided in April 1985 to reduce the number of non-prescription medicines available on the NHS, its 'limited list' included a couple of remedies that most doctors would agree are unlikely to have much if any useful pharmacological effect on the taker.
- A study carried out in the 1930s by some German doctors compared two similar groups of people suffering from warts. One group had their warts painted with what they were told was an effective wart remover, but was actually an innocuous dye that had no physical effect on the body. The other group received no treatment. Three months later, patients who had been treated with the dye had lost more of their warts than those who had been left untreated.

Taken in isolation, any one of this handful of observations

might seem unimportant, but comparable examples can be found throughout health care. There is no branch of medicine, no consultation and no type of procedure in which equally unexpected or paradoxical elements can't be found. The only conclusion to be drawn from hundreds of formal studies and thousands of anecdotes is that the tangible, material things that doctors do to and for their patients are not the sum total of the medicine they practise.

It follows that no explanation of what takes place between a patient and a health practitioner – whether orthodox or alternative – can be complete unless it takes account of the non-material elements of the process. Yet orthodox medicine consistently neglects them, and alternative medicine misunderstands or misinterprets them.

An attempt to fathom these subtle, non-material elements is intrinsically valuable, if only to grasp what is really going on when doctors, nurses, physiotherapists, acupuncturists, homeopaths, aromatherapists and all other health workers exercise their therapeutic skills. But this book has a further and wider purpose. Most people working in health care fall into one or other of two camps: the orthodox and the unorthodox. A few professionals manage to straddle both. By and large, though, we know that the men and women carrying stethoscopes and wearing white coats who pass us in the hospital corridor will be on their way to practise orthodox (scientific) medicine, while those who describe what they offer as 'natural' health care – and who probably wouldn't be found in most hospital corridors in the first place – will not. In itself this division need not matter; after all, both groups are in the business of 'pleasing' their patients. Both are trying to help those individuals overcome their illnesses, and allow them to enjoy the good health that will then follow. It's clearly in the interests of patients that the two groups co-operate. In fact their relationship is characterized not by co-operation, but by mutual mistrust and hostility.

As a medical journalist I am on the receiving end of propaganda issued by both camps. The more I read and listen, the more I realize that much of the battle is not only destructive, but futile. I am not arguing simply for mutual toleration. For either camp to tolerate those of their adversaries' remedies that they believe to be irrelevant or damaging would be lazy and negligent. Anyone who, in their opinion, sees a sick person being mistreated is bound to protest. My argument, however, is that both camps are wrong – and at the same time right. Both are building on what are really parts of the truth about health and disease; but both often behave as if their own partial truths were the whole truth.

Myths and realities

All professions have their mythologies: their idealized view of what they're doing, and why. For understandable but now outdated reasons, the greater part of medical education assumes that all health care follows broadly the same pattern. The patient develops a symptom, and visits the doctor; the doctor asks the patient questions about his or her condition, carries out a physical examination, and performs or requests whatever tests may be necessary. With all the relevant information to hand he or she then makes a diagnosis and prescribes a treatment, following which, it is hoped, the patient will recover.

Contrast this happy scenario with a comment by Dr Michael Balint, a psychiatrist whose views and ideas have done much to influence the thinking of many GPs in Britain. In an article published thirty-five years ago in the *Lancet*, he wrote:

Particularly through urbanization, a great number of people have lost their roots and connections, and large families with their complex and intimate interrelations are beginning to disappear. The individual has become more and more solitary and even lonely. If in trouble, he has hardly anyone to go to for advice, consolation, or even an opportunity to pour out his heart. He is more and more thrown back on himself. We know that in quite a number of people, perhaps in all of us, any mental or emotional stress or strain is accompanied by, or tantamount to, some bodily sensations. In such troubled states, one of the possible outlets is to drop in on one's doctor and complain.

How different is this from the idealized task described previously? Many of the patients who come to GPs are not really ill in the traditional medical sense at all. They are angry or frustrated or unhappy or without hope. They may, as Dr Balint suggests, manifest this in the form of physical symptoms; but these symptoms are not their fundamental problem. Again, the idealized consultation and diagnosis is followed by a treatment. But as infectious disease is beaten back and life expectancy increases, a growing proportion of our illnesses are of the chronic and degenerative type. These are much harder to remedy than the acute or infectious types of illness and, not surprisingly, medicine is still not so successful at dealing with them. Even when treatment is available it may have to be continued for months or years on end. At best the symptoms may be mitigated or prevented from progressing. At worst there may be unpleasant side effects and little or no improvement. The doctor becomes bored with hearing about the patient's unceasing pain and misery; the patient grows resentful that the doctor appears to have neither the skill to solve the problem nor the time to listen and sympathize.

The Office of Population Censuses and Surveys has compiled data on the number of patients suffering from particular diseases a GP with a list size of 2,500 persons might expect to see in an average year. Top of the league table are upper respiratory tract disorders (674 patients), followed by skin disorders (256). Then come chronic emotional illnesses (238 patients), pneumonia and acute bronchitis (184), acute emotional disorders (115) and chronic arthritis (111). Adding up the numbers reveals that roughly two-fifths of these patients are suffering from the kind of problems to which the 'examination-diagnosis-treatment-and-finish-with-it' model of medicine simply doesn't apply. With so much chronic anxiety, so much intractable arthritis and all the rest of it, you could even say it's a testament to GPs that many of them achieve as much as they do.

In the hope of finding something better, many patients turn to complementary medicine. But here too all is far from satisfactory – though for different reasons. The naïve patient is confronted by a bewildering variety of practitioners, some with dubious qualifications, some with none at all, some peddling the sheerest nonsense, some decrying the achievements of orthodox medicine, a few seeking only to line their own pockets. Where regulation exists there may be more than one body, each self-appointed and answerable only to its own membership. The patient who visits a practitioner may have no way of distinguishing the honest from the crooked, the eccentric or the deluded. He or she faces organizational chaos, a plethora of schools of thought (or none at all), and a paucity of objective evidence that this or that technique or therapy is likely to do any good.

Why the placebo effect?

If sick people are to get the best from everything we know about health and disease, we need a way of overcoming this sad divide. We need a way of practising medicine that melds all the partial truths into one truth: one complete understanding about human illness and how to deal with it. To achieve this happy state will require a deal of introspection, and some painful change.

There are, I'm sure, many routes towards this goal. This book will follow the path that leads from an understanding of the placebo effect – examples of which are found at the beginning of this introduction and an explanation of which will be given in chapter one. Learned accounts of its remarkable consequences have been appearing in the medical and scientific literature for decades; but, strangely, they make little impact. The placebo effect is treated as an interesting curiosity, but as little more than that. I believe that in fact it sheds a unique light on what is happening when doctor and patient – healer and would-be-healed – come together. Moreover the placebo effect in its strict definition is but one manifestation of the way in which all kinds of non-material factors – some intentional, some inadvertent – influence health. Thinking about the placebo effect offers a way of considering the destructive conflict between orthodox and complementary medicine that:

- can provide a way of understanding the origin and nature of the differences between them;
- might help them to overcome some of these differences;
- would offer the basis for an approach to health care that is no less scientific than that of orthodox medicine, and no less caring than that of complementary medicine, but is more effective than either.

When I use the phrase 'pleasing the patient', the 'pleasure' I have in mind is something more than the transient satisfactions of a good play or a well-cooked meal. Pleasure, in this context, is the state of well-being for which all of us are striving. When medicine of whatever kind helps us to attain it, we think of ourselves as having been healed. The placebo effect is a key to many insights into the nature of health and healing.

PART ONE: The Placebo Effect

1 Pink Pills and Friendly Physicians
What is the placebo effect?

Angina is a form of chest pain commonly brought on by exercise. As the heart beats faster and harder, its muscles have to do more work, so they need extra oxygen. Under normal circumstances these requirements are met by an increased flow through the coronary arteries, the small vessels that supply blood, and with it oxygen, to the heart itself. If, however, these vessels have become narrowed, they may not be able to meet the demand. For dietary or other reasons, many people have deposits of cholesterol on the lining of their arteries that cause just such a narrowing. The exercise-induced demand for additional oxygen can't be supplied and the heart is left short. The result is a pain in the chest: angina.

One of the commonest treatments for angina, a drug called glyceryl trinitrate, has been in use for over a hundred years. But this hasn't deterred doctors from searching for more effective therapies. Hormones, vitamins, cobra venom, X-rays and radioactive iodine are just a few of the many remedies that have been advocated, and then abandoned. The rise and fall of one treatment for angina, a surgical procedure, constitutes what must be one of the most thought-provoking pieces of research ever carried out in this branch of medicine.

The operation itself involved opening the patient's chest and tying off a blood vessel known as the internal mammary artery. Surgeons who began using this operation in the 1950s believed that it would increase the flow of blood through the vessels of the heart, and so cure the angina. Indeed, early reports were promising. One surgeon who had operated on thirty-five patients claimed that 'more than a third had enjoyed complete relief and there has been almost complete palliation in almost three-fourths of the group'. Another claimed that out of fifty patients who had undergone internal mammary artery ligation, some two-fifths showed objective evidence of improvement, and even more said they'd felt better following the operation. It seemed set to make a major impact on the treatment of angina.

In fact, things soon began to turn out very differently. A surgeon called Cobb enlisted seventeen patients with angina, and designed an experimental test of the operation that was more rigorous than anything previously attempted. He asked his patients to record the number of episodes of pain they experienced, and the number of tablets they required to control it. He also tested their capacity to take exercise, and measured their breathing, blood pressure and electrical activity of the heart (ECG). At the time of operation Cobb gave whichever surgeon was performing it a card telling him to do one of two things: to perform the operation as normal; or to make the necessary skin incisions, but then to sow them up again. The patient had no way of telling what had been done. After the operations some of the seventeen patients were found to have improved; but this improvement bore no relation to whether or not they had had the ligation performed. One patient, for example, who had been able to tolerate only four minutes of exercise without pain before the surgery, could manage ten minutes afterwards. Yet he was one of the group who had received the sham operation.

Although this experiment cast doubt on the value of internal mammary ligation, it was not without flaws. A more certain death blow was administered by surgeons Dimond, Kittle and Crockett. All eighteen of the patients in their study received skin incisions, but only thirteen were ligatured. Neither the patients, nor the cardiologists who subsequently assessed their progress, knew who was in which group. Ten of the thirteen patients (76 per cent) who had had the genuine operation showed a marked improvement; but so did all five who'd had the sham procedure. A 100 per cent success rate!

Following these damning results, internal mammary artery ligation disappeared from the surgical agenda. It's now thought to have no effect on the flow of blood to the heart. The affair presents a double puzzle: some patients who had had a useless operation none the less improved; and so did others who believed they'd had the operation, when, in fact, they hadn't.

Ethically speaking, these experiments are highly questionable. The patients who were chosen for the sham operation had, on the face of it, nothing to gain – and, because no operation is without risk, potentially something to lose. Indeed, a research ethics committee of the kind that nowadays scrutinizes all clinical research would probably have refused to allow such experiments. Right or wrong, though, they showed beyond any doubt that patients who believe they have received a beneficial treatment improve as a consequence. This is called the placebo effect.

Definitions

The word 'placebo' comes to us straight from the Latin for 'I shall please'. As is the way with words, its usage and precise meaning have changed over the years. A medical dictionary published in the late eighteenth century defines it as 'a commonplace method of medicine'. An early nineteenth century version has it as 'an epithet given to any medicine adopted more to please than to benefit the patient' – a definition that is inching closer towards that given in the latest edition of the *Oxford Concise Medical Dictionary*: 'a medicine that is ineffective but may help to relieve a condition because the patient has faith in its powers'.

For fine detail it's still difficult to improve on the offering of a New York physician writing 30 years ago. Dr Arthur Shapiro took a great interest in the placebo effect, and his observations are still among the most penetrating in the literature. His definition runs as follows:

Any therapeutic procedure (or that component of any therapeutic procedure) which is given deliberately to have an effect, or unknowingly has an effect on a patient, symptoms, syndrome or disease, but which is objectively without *specific* activity for the condition being treated. The therapeutic procedure may be given with or without conscious knowledge that the procedure is a placebo, may be an active (non-inert) or nonactive (inert) procedure, and includes therefore all medical procedures no matter how specific – oral and parenteral* medication, topical preparations,† inhalants, and mechanical, surgical, and psychological procedures. The placebo must be differentiated from the placebo effect which may or may not occur and which may be favourable or unfavourable. The placebo effect is defined as the changes produced by placebos.

To those with a taste for the pithy, Dr Stewart Wolf of the University of Oklahoma School of Medicine has this to offer: 'Placebo effect = any effect attributable to a pill, potion or procedure, but not to its pharmacodynamic or specific properties.'

What becomes clear from Dr Shapiro's more exhaustive definition is that the placebo effect is ubiquitous. In the example quoted earlier – the surgical procedure for dealing with angina – the manipulation of the artery couldn't of itself have brought about any useful change in the blood supply to the heart. The benefits experienced by the patients were entirely attributable to the placebo effect. However, even if the procedure itself *were* to have brought about some beneficial physiological changes, part of the improvement could still have been a placebo response. It's not a question of either/or; useless interventions may confer placebo-induced benefits; useful interventions confer specific benefits *plus* placebo benefits. So long as the

*Parenteral means administered by any route other than the mouth, e.g. by injection.
†Topical means applied directly to a part of the body, and most often the skin.

patient believes in the practitioner and his treatment, the placebo will be as much a friend to the good physician as to the quack.

As most patients have at least some faith in the skills of whatever practitioner they've chosen to consult (otherwise they presumably wouldn't be consulting him) the placebo effect has been working its healing magic for as long as sick people have sought help. In truth, many of the pills and potions dispensed by healers throughout most of history have probably been largely if not wholly useless. Which is why the history of medicine until recent times is really the history of the placebo effect itself.

Historical placebos

If you were unfortunate enough to have lived in Egypt around 1500 BC you might have been treated with lizard's blood, crocodile dung, the teeth of swine and putrid meat. Precisely how these bizarre ingredients were used to prepare a medicine is difficult to imagine. But if the effectiveness of medication really is in proportion to its unpleasantness, this brew should have been powerful stuff. A similar thought may have been in the minds of the Greek physicians who prescribed deer horn, the flesh of vipers and the spermatic fluid of frogs.

These and other such examples are quoted lovingly and at length by Arthur Shapiro, who went to great pains to comb the medical literature, ancient and modern, in search of humanity's more unlikely medicines. His searches were amply rewarded. The Roman scholar Pliny recommended eating a mouse once a month to prevent toothache. The seventh century saw Paul of Aegina using bats' blood to preserve the breasts of virgins, goats' blood for dropsy and kidney stones, domestic fowls' blood for cerebral haemorrhages, and lambs' blood for epilepsy. Until the sixteenth century, and in some cases beyond, physicians were fond of what they liked to call unicorn horn, but which was in fact powdered ivory. A remedy used in eighteenth-century Italy for curing toothache required sufferers first to crush a particular species of worm between the right thumb and forefingers, and then to touch the afflicted tooth. Remarkably, a commission that investigated these claims found that 431 out of 629 toothaches stopped immediately.

Contact with a royal person has featured throughout history as a way of curing all manner of diseases. Scrofula, a now rare form of TB, was commonly known as the King's Evil – and could be cured by the Royal Touch. Charles II alone is said to have touched more than 90,000 people. His powers don't seem to have done the King himself much good. Treating his final illness, his doctors removed a pint of blood from his right arm and half a pint from his left, gave him an emetic and an enema containing fifteen ingredients, then shaved his head and raised a blister on it. Sneezing powder was followed by more emetics and more bleeding, plus a plaster for his feet made out of pitch and pigeon dung. The doctors' final act was to give him forty drops of an extract of human skull. After this he died: a happy release.

Even men of whom one might have expected a more critical attitude to medicine seem to have gone along with a great deal of nonsense. The seventeenth-century English chemist Robert Boyle was happy to recommend a powder made of the sole of an old and much-used shoe as a way of dealing with stomach ache.

Of course, some of the less improbable among these remedies probably *did* have specific pharmacological effects. In 1785, for example, the Birmingham physician William Withering published an account of the value of an extract of foxglove in treating the water-logged tissues symptomatic of dropsy, a condition that we now recognize as resulting from heart failure. The active ingredient of this long-established folk treatment is, in fact, digitalis, chemical derivatives of which are still used to treat heart failure. Herbalists in many places and at many times have accumulated an array of plant material with all sorts of actions on the body. But practitioners whose potions tend more towards the eye-of-newt-and-skin-of-toad end of the therapeutic spectrum were largely dependent on the placebo effect for their results. It's a testament to the power of the placebo effect that all societies have been prepared to support, and even to honour, men whose medicaments were simply useless if not actually dangerous.

This is not to say that some people, more canny or more sceptical than most of their fellows, weren't suspicious about some of what was perpetrated in the name of medicine. Pierre Pomponazzi, a sixteenth-century philosopher, came very near the truth:

> We can easily conceive the marvellous effects which confidence and imagination can produce ... The cures attributed to the influence of certain relics are the effect of this imagination and confidence. Quacks and philosophers know that if the bones of any skeleton were put in place of the saint's bones, the sick would none the less experience beneficial effects if they believed that they were near veritable relics.

Progress towards the truth about many time-honoured remedies was spasmodic, and hampered by the tendency of some enthusiasts who cast out one fatuous remedy to endorse others that were just as idiotic. Paracelsus, who practised in sixteenth-century Basel, publicly burned those works of certain of his illustrious predecessors that he considered outdated, and abandoned many practices that owed more to witchcraft than to rational observation. But even his insight was patchy; he believed, for example, that certain powders applied to blood-stained garments would help to heal the injuries responsible for the stains.

Like the rest of us, doctors have always found it difficult to resist the temptation to attribute recovery from sickness to something or some event that they instinctively feel to be desirable. Many years ago the American physician Edward Trudeau, believing himself to be dying of TB, went up into the Adirondack Mountains to spend what he thought would be his remaining weeks. In fact, he recovered. This he attributed to the healing properties of mountain air, and so gave support to the widespread but insupportable belief that mountain air is a cure for this disease. 'He might with equal justification,' one critic has remarked, 'have credited the nourishing qualities of the rabbits which he shot on the hillside.'

One of the first and most explicit statements of the non-material element in the effect of medical potions came from an American doctor called Quimby, writing in the late 1850s. 'Through a great many mistakes, and the prescription of a great many useless drugs, I was led to re-examine the question, and came in the end to the position I now hold: the cure does not depend upon any drug, but simply in the patient's belief in the doctor or the medicine.'

Dr Arthur Shapiro's researches into the medical literature have shown that relatively little was published on the placebo effect during the first half of the present century. One magnificent exception was a 1920 book on *Medicine, Magic and Religion* by William Rivers. Arthur Shapiro quotes him with approval:

The action of suggestion can never be excluded in any form of medical treatment, whether it be explicitly designed to act upon the mind or whether ostensibly it is purely physical in character ... If we confine our attention to our own culture, it is only within the last fifty or sixty years that there has been any clear recognition of the vast importance of the mental factor in the production and treatment of disease, and even now this knowledge is far from being fully recognized either by the profession or the laity.

And, looking back, he adds:

Few can now be found who will deny that the success which attended the complex prescriptions, and most of the dietetic remedies of the last generation, was due mainly if not entirely to the play of faith and suggestion.

Universal influence

Documented studies of the placebo effect have ranged over all manner of disorders, including rheumatoid arthritis, hay fever, headache, pain, ulcers, high blood pressure, anxiety, depression, schizophrenia, colds and sea sickness. If the placebo effect is indeed a universal phenomenon operating in conjunction with all remedies – useful and otherwise – the list could, presumably, be extended indefinitely.

Let's return to the treatment of angina for a further example of the placebo effect at work. Just over ten years ago two American doctors, Herbert Benson and David McCallie, reviewed the efficacy of five treatments for angina. One, the ligaturing of the internal mammary artery, has already been described. One other is also surgical; the other three are drug treatments.

Methyl xanthines are a group of chemical agents that were thought, back in the 1920s, to overcome angina by dilating the coronary arteries, thus allowing more blood to reach the heart. One study, for example, found a moderate to marked improvement in half to three-quarters of the patients studied. But neither these nor other researchers used a comparison or control group of patients against whom to assess the changes wrought by the drug. The rigorous protocols nowadays used for assessing medicines (to be described in the next chapter), which would have prevented such misleading conclusions, were not yet routine.

The xanthines began to fall from favour in the 1930s when two groups of researchers reassessed them, this time using placebo pills as a comparison. In both cases, between 30 and 40 per cent of patients improved, irrespective of whether they had received xanthine or placebo.

Much the same fate befell another drug called khellin, introduced in the 1940s. Early studies claimed between 70 and 90 per cent effectiveness – but within ten years more sceptical accounts began to be published. Once again it was the use of proper control groups of patients that revealed the weakness of the previous claims. Vitamin E, the third of the drugs reviewed by Drs Benson and McCallie, likewise attracted supporters and then lost them.

The other surgical procedure for angina also involved the internal mammary artery. Instead of ligaturing it, the surgeon would implant it into a 3–4 centimetre tunnel cut into the wall of the heart. The hope was to establish a new circulation that would once again bring extra blood to it. This technique was introduced in the 1950s, and became popular in the 1960s. Despite impressive claims of both subjective and objective improvement, enthusiasm for the procedure eventually waned. Yet before it was abandoned between 10,000 and 15,000 of these operations were carried out – with roughly one in every twenty patients dying as a result of the procedure itself.

As Benson and McCallie observe, there has been a pattern to these events: one that seems to recur each time someone dreams up a new but, as is later established, ineffective treatment. First there is anecdotal evidence. Then comes a series of inadequate trials organized by enthusiastic doctors. Later more sceptical investigators take the trouble to devise more searching assessments. Finally, it becomes clear that most of the benefit results as a consequence of the placebo effect – and the treatment is abandoned. There is more to be said about this question of enthusiastic versus sceptical doctors. But first, a little more on the character of the placebo effect – and in particular on one of its most celebrated manifestations: the colour of the pill.

Rainbow colours

Twenty years ago, three psychiatrists and a statistician working in Newcastle decided to examine the possible influence of tablet colour on the effectiveness of treatments for anxiety. The drug they used was oxazepam, a minor tranquillizer belonging to the same group as Valium. They had the tablets made up in three colours: green, yellow and red. The subjects were forty-eight patients, all with normal colour vision, diagnosed as suffering from anxiety.

The researchers used two methods of measuring the severity of the patients' symptoms. One was a self-rating method in which each person taking part was asked to use his or her own words to describe the main symptoms: 'feeling afraid', 'palpitations', 'low in spirits' or whatever. The symptoms were then written on a score card, and the patient graded the severity of each on a continuous scale ranging from absent through moderate to very severe. Each patient spent one week on each colour tablet, allocated in random order, and repeated their self-assessment every evening. The doctors, too, graded each patient's symptoms at the beginning of the experiment, and at weekly intervals thereafter.

The patients were told only that the tablets had all been found to help others with their condition, and that the aim of the study was to find which of the three kinds was most effective in relieving their particular symptoms. The results showed that anxiety responded best to green colour pills, while symptoms of depression responded best to yellow.

Although this is one of the studies most often quoted to illustrate the placebo effect, its main findings were only trends. They did not reach statistical significance. In other words, there was a possibility that the apparent influence of colour might actually have been due to some other factor or simply to chance. A less well known but more impressive demonstration of the effect of colour was published a couple of years later. The subjects in this case were not sick people, but healthy medical students; indeed its perpetrators, three doctors at the University of Cincinnati College of Medicine, used it to teach students about the importance of non-drug factors in prescribing.

The organizers asked each of a class of medical students to take part in a study of two drugs, one a stimulant the other a sedative. The students were told that each could have both physiological and psychological effects, some beneficial and some adverse. They were given examples of what to expect: a change in pupil size or pulse rate; or a tendency to become cheerful and talkative, or drowsy and sluggish. Each student received a pill, chosen at random, which was either pink or blue. They weren't told which pills were stimulants and which sedatives – or rather which pills were *supposed* to be which, because all were in fact placebos. Having swallowed the pills and given them time to work, the students assessed and recorded their responses.

As far as psychological changes were concerned, all but three out of a group of fifty-six reported changes. On the adverse side, more than half said they felt drowsy. The commonest beneficial effect, experienced by more than a third, was a sense of being more relaxed and less jittery. Physiological changes included pulse rate (up in 66 per cent, down in 15 per cent) and blood pressure (down in 71 per cent, up in 18 per cent). The students also described a range of other side effects including headaches, dizziness and difficulty in concentrating.

The influence of the colour of the pills was clear. Two-thirds of those who had taken blue pills felt they had become less alert, but only a quarter who had taken pink pills felt this way. Three-quarters of those who had taken blue pills felt more drowsy, but only a third who had taken pink. In short, although all the pills were inert, blue was associated with a sedative action, pink with a stimulant one – and once the pills had been taken, the students' minds and bodies responded accordingly.

Red to kill the pain

Definitive proof of the importance of colour when using placebos given not to healthy medical students, but to real patients with real illnesses came in 1974. Dr Edward Huskisson of St Bartholomew's Hospital in London organized a complicated three-part study of the treatment of arthritis using simple analgesics such as aspirin and paracetamol. One arm of the experiment compared the effectiveness of three analgesics and a placebo. Different patients were given tablets of different colours: yellow, blue, green and red. Predictably, all three active drugs, irrespective of colour, gave better pain relief than the placebo preparations considered as a group. The most intriguing finding came when the results were re-analysed to compare the various coloured placebos individually. Red was most effective at relieving pain, followed by blue, green and yellow. Red placebos were so powerful that their capacity to dull the pain of arthritis almost equalled that of the active drugs! It seems strange that drug manufacturers have taken so little notice of this finding. Perhaps they feel it's cheating to sell analgesics that rely for their effect on something other than pharmacology!

It is not only colour that influences our preconceptions about medicines, and so their value. In 1981, Branthwaite and Cooper, two psychologists at the University of Keele, studied the effects of branding on the power of aspirin to relieve headaches. Aspirin can be bought in one of two forms: as unbranded, generic tablets; or in one of many branded formulations, with or without other ingredients, in packs that are often made familiar through advertising. At the time this study was done, roughly two-thirds of analgesics sold were in branded form – which, of course, cost more.

Branthwaite and Cooper recruited more than 800 women who claimed to use painkillers for a headache at least once a month, and allocated them at random to four different groups. Women in two of the groups each received fifty tablets packed in a cannister identical to those used to supply one of the most popular branded analgesics on the market. The tablets were marked with the manufacturer's name. The other two groups were given unmarked tablets in plain cannisters. One each of the branded and unbranded groups was given aspirin, and the other dummy pills identical in appearance.

When the results were collected, both types of aspirin tablet proved – as one would expect – to be more effective at relieving the pain of headaches than placebo tablets. But the branded aspirin was more effective than the unbranded aspirin, and the branded placebo was more effective than the unbranded placebo. 'In relative terms,' say the authors, 'the pharmacologically active ingredients would appear to account for some two-thirds to three-quarters of the pain relief, and branding for one-quarter to one-third, over and above that obtained with the unbranded placebo.' In short, the widespread belief that branded preparations are more effective is a self-fulfilling prophesy – even though, pharmacologically speaking, it is groundless.

The Keele experimenters weren't the first to try measuring the placebo effect. Back in 1955, Dr Henry Beecher of Harvard Medical School in Massachusetts reported that in studies of severe post-operative pain he and his colleagues had consistently found that 30 per cent of patients get relief from a placebo. He averaged out the success rate of placebos in fifteen studies involving more than a thousand patients suffering not only from post-operative pain, but also from a variety of other conditions ranging from angina to seasickness. The figure he came up with was 35.2 per cent, plus or minus 2.3 per cent. The validity of this mathematical averaging is questionable. But a glance at the figures presented in all fifteen studies is enough to see that most do fall in the 30–40 per cent range. So Dr Beecher's comment on the results is justified: 'The constancy of the placebo effect ... in a fairly wide variety of conditions, including pain, nausea and mood changes, suggests that a fundamental mechanism in common is operating in these several cases ...' It's a thought I'll be returning to in the next chapter.

'Nocebo' effects

Not all placebo effects are beneficial. That they mostly are is because patients don't usually go to the doctor believing that what he'll prescribe is likely to do them harm. A hint that placebos can, however, have negative as well as positive effects is apparent in the student experiment. Some of them, you may remember, were warned of the possibility of adverse effects from the pink and blue tablets; and some of them duly experienced those effects. In his studies of the placebo treatment of people suffering from post-operative pain Dr Henry Beecher of Boston recorded thirty-five different side effects, including nausea, dry mouth, headaches, difficulty in concentrating and fatigue.

In so far as this is the placebo phenomenon, but working

against the patient rather than *for* him, a different word is used: the 'nocebo' effect, this too drawn from Latin (*noceo*, meaning to injure or do harm).

A striking instance of what one can only describe as the placebo and nocebo effects operating simultaneously was reported in 1969 in the *British Journal of Psychiatry*. A doctor working in Prague described his dealings with a forty-four-year-old woman suffering from schizophrenia. She had been treated with several standard drugs – none of which had brought her illness fully under control. At some time during 1963, the doctor who had been looking after her decided to try prescribing a placebo: a drug that he described to her as 'a new major tranquillizer without any side effects'. Unlike any of the previous drugs she'd taken, this seemed to work, and from that time until 1967 she remained well and able to work.

In the summer of 1967, perhaps as a consequence of being given a more responsible job, she began to develop headaches, anxiety, insomnia and some hints of her previous schizophrenic symptoms. Her response to this was to increase the number of tablets she took daily from three to nine to twelve. Events came to a head in December of that year. The woman was unable to work, and spent her time pacing up and down her room. She couldn't think properly, and was sweating profusely. She eventually confessed that having upped her daily consumption of pills to twenty-five she had run out, and hadn't had one for two days.

With the woman's agreement her doctor wrote to her employer suggesting that she not be given the new job. The employer agreed, the woman felt able to return to work, and her consumption of the placebo pills dropped back to two per day.

Commenting on the case, the doctor who reported it (Oldrich Vinar of Prague's Psychiatric Research Institute) points out that his patient showed all the characteristics of drug dependency. She had a compulsive desire to take the tablets; she kept increasing the dose; she couldn't stop taking them without the help of a psychiatrist; and her symptoms on being deprived of her pills were not unlike those of a withdrawal reaction. All this – the beneficial effects *and* the adverse – brought about by pills that were pharmacologically inactive!

Because the placebo effect depends on a subtle influence of mind over body, it is reasonable to wonder if some people might be more susceptible to it than others – if there is, indeed, such a person as a typical 'placebo reactor', perhaps someone who is more than averagely suggestible. In at least one experiment, standard tests of suggestibility showed little correlation with a tendency to respond to placebos. Personality, too, has been a popular theme in attempts to characterize responders. They've been described as more neurotic, compliant, religious, anxious, and hypochondriacal, and as less educated. But the results of most such analyses have proved contradictory. So have attempts to define responders by sex and age. The terms 'placebo responder' and 'placebo non-responder' seem to have little value except in describing the result of any one experiment.

In all probability, anyone can respond to a placebo, given the appropriate setting and circumstances. So what is it that mobilizes the placebo effect? Among the most important factors are the doctor, and his or her relationship with the patient.

The doctor as placebo

Doctors first contemplated their own potency as agents of healing long before anyone began thinking in terms of placebo effects. The Roman physician Galen is supposed to have remarked of his profession that, 'He cures most in whom most are confident'. In our own century we have the psychiatrist Michael Balint, a man whose ideas on the relationship between doctors and patients have influenced many in the profession, especially GPs. In an article published in 1955 in the *Lancet* under the title 'The doctor, his patient, and the illness', he recalls a seminar held at London's Tavistock Clinic where he worked:

PINK PILLS AND FRIENDLY PHYSICIANS

In one of these seminars the first topic discussed was the drugs usually prescribed by the practitioner. Very soon the discussion revealed – not for the first time – that by far the most frequently used drug in general practice was *the doctor himself*. It was not only the medicine in the bottle or the pills in the box which mattered, but also the way the doctor gave them to his patient – in fact the whole atmosphere in which the drug was given and taken.

A persuasive demonstration of this claim was forthcoming one year later when a doctor working in Kansas investigated the varying degrees of success with which his colleagues used the then relatively new major tranquillizer chlorpromazine. Even when treating similar groups of patients under similar circumstances, the results often differed quite markedly. Suspecting that the attitudes of the staff might account for at least some of the variation, Dr Paul Feldman devised an experiment involving more than 300 patients suffering from schizophrenia or schizophrenic-type illnesses. Their treatment was supervised by twenty-seven doctors, each of whom Dr Feldman placed into one of four categories, depending on their attitude towards chlorpromazine.

Doctors in category one were wholeheartedly enthusiastic about the new drug. Category two comprised the moderately conservative majority: 'Let's try it and see'. In category three were doctors who were openly sceptical about the drug but prepared to try it. Category four doctors rejected this form of treatment, and refused to use it.

Excluding the last category, Dr Feldman found that the more enthusiastic the doctors were about the treatment they were prescribing, the better their results.

It seems likely that the placebo effect originates not so much in the act of swallowing the pill as in the interaction between patient and doctor that precedes it. Going to see a doctor can of itself be therapeutic – with some consequent embarrassment when the patient tries to explain why the toothache that was so unbearable three hours ago has mysteriously vanished. Simply removing patients from the environment that they associate with sickness can also be beneficial. But what happens from the moment the patient enters the consulting room and sits facing the doctor seems to be crucial.

Arthur Shapiro offers this analysis:

The interested doctor who imparts confidence, who is friendly and reassuring to patients, who performs a thorough examination, and who is not anxious, conflicted or guilty about the patient or his treatment is more likely to elicit positive placebo reactions. Negative placebo reactions are more likely when the doctor is angry, rejecting, and contemptuous towards patients or seriously preoccupied with his own problems.

In the next paragraph he continues:

The doctor's attitude towards the treatment is an ingredient compounded into every prescription ... Although a placebo may be as effective as an active drug when the doctor's attitude towards the treatment is negative, the active drug is significantly better than the placebo when the doctor's attitude towards the treatment is positive.

When some doctors speak of the art of medicine, they do so for reasons that are wholly self-serving. Their proclaimed 'art' is no more than a smokescreen behind which to hide their reluctance to evaluate what they do and, if necessary, alter it. But reading those passages quoted from Shapiro gives a legitimate meaning to the phrase 'art of medicine'. Like many arts, those of medicine can be taught; but there will always be individuals who seem to need no lessons in the skills of putting people at ease, talking simply and lucidly, and inspiring confidence. Happy the patients who have such physicians.

Readers with a taste for unnecessary neologisms will be pleased to know that there is now a term to describe the phenomenon of doctor-aroused placebo effects. It is 'iatroplacebogenesis', derived from the Greek *iatrikos*, meaning a healer. Having mentioned the word we can now forget it. The concept, though, is important – and one reviewer makes an interesting distinction between directly- and indirectly-aroused placebo effects.

The direct form is the more obvious. The doctor makes it

clear that he is interested in the patient's well-being, and the patient responds positively to this knowledge – with the beneficial consequences already described. Indirect arousal of the placebo effect occurs when the patient realizes that the doctor's interest is not primarily in him or herself, but in some interesting or unusual facet of the illness. Conventional wisdom would suggest that this is not a good thing, and in many cases, no doubt, the patient does suffer accordingly.

Alternatively, and certainly more encouragingly, the patient, having perceived that the doctor is paying exceptional attention to the ailment, is prompted to feel great confidence in that doctor. This, no doubt, is why the investigation of an illness (as opposed to its treatment) may by itself prove beneficial!

Schizophrenics in one special research unit, for example, were found to undergo an 80 per cent improvement, even though receiving no extra treatment. There's a close analogy here with what is known as the 'Hawthorne effect'. This was named after the factory in which it was found that the increased attention paid to workers while their efficiency was being studied actually boosted that efficiency.

More evidence of the importance of doctors' attitudes comes from a number of studies that have shown that patients benefit more from drug therapy when doctors themselves anticipate that they will do so. In the late 1970s a couple of American oral surgeons, Steven Gryll and Martin Katahn, looked at this in more detail. They took as their example an attempt to reduce fear and pain in patients about to receive an injection of dental anaesthetic. Each subject was given a pill, and told either that it had an excellent track record in minimizing pain, or that it only worked for some people, but was worth a try anyway. Some staff were instructed to deliver this information in a warm and friendly manner; others to do so coldly and impersonally.

The results showed that patients who had received the more positive message felt less anxiety before the injection, and experienced less pain. They also rated the pain as less intense when the information was delivered in a friendly manner.

Differences of enthusiasm arousing greater or lesser placebo responses may account for a phenomenon noted many times, and referred to earlier in the context of surgery for angina: the tendency of worthless treatments to give good results when first introduced. Dr Henry Beecher of Boston has divided the various surgeons who published their findings on internal mammary artery ligation for angina into two categories: enthusiasts and sceptics. In total, the enthusiasts achieved 38 per cent total relief of pain; the corresponding figure for the sceptics was only 10 per cent! Beecher also quotes figures from thirty years ago for a now discredited form of surgery used to treat duodenal ulcers. One surgeon, an enthusiast for the procedure, reported that 82 per cent of his patients were still free of ulcers five years after the operation. Another surgeon, sceptical of its benefits, declared that the figure for his patients was only 47 per cent. Reading these figures, one looks nervously at the exploits of today's surgeons, every bit as enthusiastic as were their predecessors about their cherished procedures.

Of course, it could be argued that if the placebo effect has worked, and the patient is much improved, why worry? The pitfall here is that removal from the circumstances that serve to generate and reinforce the placebo effect – being visited daily by a highly enthusiastic surgeon, for example – will lead to its disappearance. In principle, no doubt, placebo effects can be maintained indefinitely, but circumstances are seldom such that this is likely to happen. So while placebo effects are to be welcomed, it is as well to be able to distinguish them from specific pharmacologically or physiologically induced changes in the body. And this, of course, necessitates the creation of an elaborate research methodology.

2 A Tiresome Distraction
The placebo effect in medical research

As far as most medical researchers are concerned, the placebo effect represents but one thing: a nuisance to be dispensed with. To understand why they take this view, it's necessary to appreciate the nature of the task they're undertaking.

The earliest forms of scientific endeavour were largely descriptive. The hope was that the facts would, by their very accumulation, reveal patterns that made sense of what was otherwise mysterious. Description, though, has its limits. Hence the invention of more interventionist or experimental methods of investigation. As far as living things are concerned, the most basic of these is dissection. Aristotle was the first to make extensive use of it in studying animals – though not humans. Peering into the hidden parts of an organism is a necessary first step towards understanding how it works. But appearances alone are misleading. Aristotle, for example, thought that the purpose of the lungs was to cool the region around the heart.

Even more valuable to science than systematically dismembering the biological or physical system being investigated is to disturb it in some way, and see how it responds. In modern science this idea is taken for granted. As a simple example, take the iris of the eye. Just as the aperture in front of a camera lens can be adjusted to regulate the amount of light falling on the film, so the iris of the eye alters the diameter of the pupil and increases or reduces the light reaching the retina. But simply looking at the iris under constant illumination reveals nothing.

Only when you 'disturb' the system – by brightening or dimming the light – do you see the iris at work, and begin to form an idea of its natural function. A great deal of experimental science is an elaboration of this simple idea.

By comparison with physics and chemistry, biology was slow to adopt this more active approach to the pursuit of knowledge. It continued to be dominated by the natural historians who were primarily interested in collecting, describing and classifying their material. Form held more attractions for them than function. Think of the Victorian enthusiasm for museums filled with exotic creatures that had been hunted down, killed, crated up and despatched home from all parts of the globe to be lovingly stuffed or pickled, mounted in glass boxes or jars, labelled in elegant copperplate, and then displayed on rows of fine mahogany shelving. It is an indication of the priorities of many if not most biologists.

All attempts to acquire knowledge have their own pitfalls. One of the earliest observations was the simple and obvious fact that the Sun travels around the Earth. Experience seemed to offer a daily confirmation of its movement. But experience was misleading, and what seemed simple and obvious happened not to be as it appeared. The realization that the Earth, in fact, went round the Sun was a truth long in dawning, and both emotionally and intellectually difficult to accept.

Another trap for the unwary lies in the failure to distinguish between association and causation. The fact that two things repeatedly happen at the same time doesn't mean that one is necessarily a consequence of the other. Both may be the result of some third event of which the observer is unaware. To avoid these and dozens of other such intellectual quagmires, science has imposed upon itself a set of elaborate and sometimes tedious but none the less essential safeguards. Researchers are required not only to publish their findings, but also to describe their methods in sufficient detail to allow others to repeat the work. Indeed, the repeatability of an experiment is one of the criteria by which scientists judge the claims of their peers.

Medical research

Medical research is now part of this enterprise. This is not to say that the *practice* of medicine has yet become anything like as scientific as its propagandists might have you believe. But the introduction of scientific rigour has helped to rid doctoring of some of the guesswork, prejudice and mythology that have dominated much of its history.

As in other branches of learning, medicine's first attempts at acquiring new knowledge relied on observation and description. Back in the fourth century BC, Hippocrates kept detailed casenotes about many of his patients. He described their appearance, their fevers, their behaviour and the nature of their urine and stools. He noted such matters as their work and where they lived, and he even tried to relate their illnesses to the climate and to other features of the environment. It is a testament to the enduring value of this approach that many of today's medical journals still include a section devoted to 'clinical observations' or 'case histories'. These accounts are more sophisticated than the records kept by Hippocrates, but in essence they are much the same. Generations of doctors have read these descriptions and, through them, learned how better to recognize disease in their own patients. Case histories may offer valuable hints about treatment or prognosis and, as they accumulate, they make it possible to distinguish the exceptions and oddities from what are the first glimmerings of a new pattern of disease.

In this context it's worth recalling a modest publication called *Mortality and Morbidity Weekly*. Issued by the Center for Disease Control in Atlanta, Georgia, this journal reports not only on epidemics of disease, but also on small clusters or even individual cases. The edition of 5 June 1981 carried a brief two-page article headed 'Pneumocystis pneumonia – Los Angeles'. Its authors described the case histories of five young men, all active homosexuals, who'd been treated for this relatively rare form of pneumonia at three different hospitals between October 1980 and May 1981. Two of them had died. The closing paragraph of the report includes the following words: 'All the above observations suggest the possibility of a cellular-immune dysfunction related to a common exposure that predisposes individuals to opportunistic infections . . .'

As you may have guessed, this report – written as a series of case-notes followed by some speculative comment – was one of the first sirens alerting doctors to the emergence of the disease we now call AIDS. Rightly, then, description continues to hold an important place in medicine.

Accounts of this kind are essentially anecdotal. Indeed anecdote plays a useful role in medical advance; it is the raw material that inspires new theories, and new lines of investigation. But the problem with anecdotal evidence is that, by definition, it is incomplete. To generalize from personal experience of half a dozen cases in which giving this or that drug seemed to have this or that beneficial effect is dangerous. Maybe the half dozen were unusual; maybe doctor and patients were plain lucky.

If living organisms were as uniform in performance and as predictable in behaviour as machines, biomedical research would be straightforward. Check the performance date of the engine in the handbook, make whatever adjustment is being considered, run the engine again, and measure its new performance. If the figures improve: good. If they fall, then back to the drawing-board. The variability of biological systems makes such simple testing impossible. In all their characteristics – muscle strength, speed of digestion, reaction time, kidney function, bowel movements, blink rate – living things show a spectrum of activity. And their performance varies not only between one individual and another but also from day to day within each individual.

The need for large numbers

Better by far, then, to find out what happens not just to six patients, but to 600. It is this attempt to pool the findings from large numbers of people, and so reach conclusions that should be more generally applicable, that led to the development of what are referred to in medicine as 'trials'. If, on balance, the majority of the 600 patients taking a medicine benefit from it, then so should the majority of the next 6,000 or 600,000 who take the drug when it becomes more widely available. To market it to that number on the evidence derived from just six people would be little short of reckless.

But the need to test a new drug or a new procedure on large numbers of subjects is merely the first of the conditions that have to be met. How do you know that the drug is doing them good? By what yardstick is this judgement to be made?

Suppose you develop a drug to treat a disease for which there is no existing therapy. Having recruited suitable volunteers, you give them the drug and see what happens. A week later you find that three-quarters of them have greatly improved. Does that mean the drug is effective? Not necessarily. A great deal of illness is self-limiting; it clears up of its own accord. So how can you be sure that most if not all of these patients wouldn't have got better without your treatment?

The procedure necessary to answer this question is the controlled trial. Among a group of patients all suffering from the same illness, half are treated and half are not. If there is no existing treatment, and no certainty that the new treatment will do any good (it might even do harm), there is no ethical dilemma about withholding it from half the subjects. If those who took the drug do better than those who didn't take it, can we now be certain that the drug is helpful?

Once again we can't – this time on account of the placebo effect. The researcher knows that when people take a drug that they believe – or at least hope – will cure them, it will have at least some beneficial action: the placebo response. To discover if the new drug really does have any useful specific action on the body over and above the placebo effect, the researcher must make his trial slightly more elaborate. To discount the placebo effect, he must make sure that even those subjects who don't take the drug take something that they believe will, or at least might, help them. They must take a dummy pill, identical in size, shape, colour and taste to those pills that contain the active ingredient. Under this arrangement, everyone taking part in the study will then be subject to the placebo effect, but only half the subjects will also get the specific pharmacological effects of the drug itself. As long as none of the patients know which type of pill they're getting, their own expectations can't bias the results. Any extra improvement in the group taking the active pill must be due to the specific action of its ingredients.

But who is to get the drug, and who the dummy pill? Can we afford to let the doctor in charge of the experiment choose? The answer has to be no because the doctor will, naturally enough, be tempted to give the active pills to those patients who seem to be sicker. Hence the development of trials in which subjects are allocated active or dummy pills entirely at random.

Under this arrangement, the patient doesn't know whether he or she is getting active or dummy pills, but the doctor does have this information. Is this acceptable? The answer, yet again, has to be no. There may be something in the doctor's manner when he or she hands patients what he or she knows are the dummy pills: some tiny lack of conviction that the patient may, almost subconsciously, detect and respond to. If the patient has slightly less faith in the dummy pills, and the placebo effect is just that little bit less powerful, the value of the trial will have been undermined. And what happens when the doctor re-examines the patients to look for evidence of benefit from the new drug? If the doctor is keen to show that the new treatment is effective, he'll naturally hope to find that those who took the active pill are doing better than those who didn't. His judgement may be less than objective.

The way around this source of bias is to ensure that neither patient *nor* doctor knows who took which pill. Which pills are active and which are dummies is known only to a third party who keeps this secret until all patients have been assessed and the experiment is over.

This 'double-blind controlled trial', as it is known, has

become the gold standard for much medical research. Superficially it appears to suggest that neither doctors nor their patients can be trusted to know their own minds and reach objective judgements. But it is not dishonesty that these rather cumbersome arrangements are designed to guard against. The enemy is subconscious bias – and the placebo effect. From the point of view of the medical researcher endeavouring to discover if a new drug really does offer benefits, the placebo effect is indeed a tiresome distraction.

So what is the basis for this ubiquitous and, away from research, helpful phenomenon?

3 The Healing Mind
The mechanism of the placebo effect

People unfamiliar with the placebo effect are sometimes puzzled to learn that the colour of a pill may be significant, or that patients often respond to a medicine that, unknown to them, is completely inert. Surprise does at first seem to be in order when hearing of something so apparently outlandish. But reflection drives one to the opposite conclusion: that it would be far more surprising if the placebo effect did not exist.

By and large, things do not happen to our bodies simply because we wish them to. If I cut my finger I cannot will the blood vessels instantly to close down, or the wound to heal within five minutes. If I catch measles I cannot expect the spots to disappear overnight simply because I want them to. The lesson of daily experience appears to be that our minds have no great influence over our bodies – and for much of the time we behave as if they have none at all. Yet if we put disease to one side, and instead consider the ordinary everyday relationship between our state of mind and what happens in our bodies, we soon realize that any notion of a separation is entirely false.

By thinking of something sad, we can make our eyes shed tears; by imagining erotic images, men can give themselves erections and women start to secrete fluid into their vaginas; thinking of someone hated or feared will make the heart beat more rapidly; consciously telling a lie will induce a tiny increase in the amount of sweat being secreted on to the surface of the skin. None of the causes of these responses need have any material reality; the hater doesn't have to be in the presence of the hated, and the ideal man or woman provoking the sexual fantasy need not exist. Yet the states of mind they induce result in material changes within the body. These and other equally obvious examples illustrate the capacity of the mind to influence the body.

Given the ubiquity of this phenomenon, it would be surprising if such effects were to play no part in shaping our health or altering the progress of our diseases. The placebo effect is merely one such influence of mind on body – and if surprise *is* still appropriate, it should be not so much at the existence of the effect as over its subtlety and magnitude.

Speculating on mechanisms

How the placebo effect works is still a matter of speculation. Clearly it starts with the patient's belief, conscious or otherwise, that what the doctor has to offer will be beneficial. In purely materialist terms, a belief about something can be thought of as a particular state of mind. And, equally materialistically, a state of mind exists in the brain as a particular pattern of organization within a particular part of it. This pattern could take the form of a distribution of certain chemicals within or between specific cells; it could be encoded electrically, as an array of charges across a membrane; or it might even be represented as a series of structural modifications in a set of cell membranes. All these things are conceptually plausible. What *is* actually happening – how a memory is stored or a thought activated – we do not know. But the existence of computers – even simple devices such as the word processor on which I'm typing this book – demonstrates that vast quantities of information can be stored in small spaces by organizing the substance of the storage medium in some specified manner.

Mind, on this view, is an emergent property: the outcome of highly complex and constantly changing patterns of organization encoded within matter. And having made this jump from mind to matter, it becomes easier to consider – again conceptually – how a change in what we think, feel or believe can precipitate a material change in some part of the body. Computer analogies usually describe the brain as the hardware, and the mind as the software or instructions for manipulating the information stored within it. We don't find it surprising or mysterious that a change to the electronic pattern within a computer's memory (instructing it to print a document, for example) effects a physical change (the actual printing of the document). Perhaps it should be equally unsurprising that a change to those states of mind that represent 'confidence' or 'optimism' or 'faith' can manifest themselves as physiological changes in pain suppression, wound healing or the effectiveness of our immune defence mechanisms.

The opiates within

Given a plan of the brain and nervous system, a list of the body's hormones and their functions, an elemental knowledge of human physiology, and unbounded licence to use the imagination, it's possible (and entertaining) to devise all sorts of plausible explanations of the placebo phenomenon. There is, however, one explanation that is not only plausible, but also rooted in experimental evidence. It is based on the actions of a group of chemicals found naturally in the body: the endorphins.

For thousands of years, humans have used an extract of the opium poppy, *Papaver somniferum*, as an analgesic. Besides dulling pain, it induces a feeling of warmth and tranquillity. But it also has distinct drawbacks: it's addictive and it may induce nausea, lethargy, and violent changes of mood. Refining the ingredients of opium gives us morphine, still widely used in medicine. Further chemical processing yields diamorphine, more often known as heroin: an even more effective pain-killer. Collectively these and other related drugs are called opiates; and the natural versions such as morphine are now outnumbered by synthetic equivalents such as methadone and pethidine.

A world without opiates would be a world in which pain was harder to avoid; they do indeed seem to be a gift of nature. But what is it about these molecules – *plant* molecules, remember – that allows them to have such a potent effect on humans? The answer came in the mid-1970s when two American researchers, Solomon Snyder and Candace Pert, discovered that the surfaces of many cells bear a type of molecule called an opiate receptor.

The idea of receptors wasn't in itself new. Nor indeed was the notion of opiate receptors in particular; their existence had been predicted several years previously. The importance of the receptor concept lies in the way in which it allowed biologists to understand why hormones, neurotransmitters (the chemical messages by which adjacent nerve cells communicate with one another), and certain drugs are able to exert such a specific influence on the body. An injection of the hormone insulin, for example, alters the recipient's physiology in such a way that the amount of glucose present in the blood will fall. The male hormone testosterone, on the other hand, promotes muscle growth, male behaviour, and the physical attributes of masculinity. There is complete specificity in these effects. Female diabetics do not have to lie awake at night worrying that their bodies may mistake injected insulin for testosterone and cause them to start sprouting moustaches! The basis of this specificity is the receptor system.

Imagine the receptor on the surface of a cell as being a lock. Inserting the appropriate key and turning it will activate certain events within that cell. The outcome of those events might – to stick to the examples used already – be a fall in blood sugar, or the initiation of some aspect of male behaviour. Whatever the outcome, it represents something that the body must do – but not all the time. Hence the need for switches to bring about these events when required, and for keys able to unlock these switches. The insulin molecule is one such key, the testosterone molecule another. Hormones such as these are produced by the body – usually in a particular gland – when a certain outcome is required: an adjustment of blood sugar, say. The hormone enters the bloodstream, circulates around the body, and eventually reaches its target cells, the ones that must make the response. The locks on these cells, the receptors, are constructed in such a way that only molecules with a very specific shape will fit into them. As soon as the appropriate molecule comes along, and does fit, the receptor will be switched on, so initiating the required process.

To demonstrate the existence of opiate receptors, Snyder and Pert used a then fairly new drug called naloxone. This is an opiate antagonist: a chemical that tends to reverse the effects brought about by morphine and other drugs of the opiate family. Using morphine, and also naloxone that had been radioactively-labelled (and could therefore be traced once it had been administered) the two researchers were able to show that these agents competed for the same sites of attachment within the body. When they administered a dose of morphine, they found that a certain proportion would stick to the receptors. But if the morphine was preceded by a dose of naloxone, less morphine would stick inside the body. The explanation had to be that the naloxone was binding itself to the opiate receptors, and preventing the attachment of any morphine that subsequently appeared.

The existence of opiate receptors provided a very satisfactory explanation for the swift and powerful effect of opiate drugs on the body. But it also created another puzzle: why should the body have a system apparently designed to respond to a group of chemicals extracted from plants? Did it really make sense to imagine the body's opiate receptors sitting there on cell surfaces throughout the body, doing nothing until the day when that individual chanced to take a dose of heroin or pethidine? Clearly it did not. The explanation for the existence of opiate receptors had to be that the body makes its own opiate drugs: natural variants of morphine. This tantalizing thought sent a number of researchers in pursuit of such substances and the race was won by John Hughes and Hans Kosterlitz of the University of Aberdeen. They found a small molecule they named enkephalin; the first of the natural opiates to be identified.

Further research led to the discovery of other molecules in this category, the group as a whole acquiring the name 'endorphins', a contraction of 'endogenous morphines'. But, once again, solving this puzzle created yet another: for what purpose does the body make and respond to natural opiates? In view of the effect that morphine has on the body, the first guess is still the best one: that endorphins have a part to play in modulating our perception of pain.

Natural pain-killers

Unpleasant as pain may be, it does have an essential function. It indicates forcefully that all is not well with the body, and acts as a stimulus to do something to remedy the problem. However, there are occasions when pain is redundant. Following traumatic injury – the severing of a limb, for example – it is not necessary to rely on a burst of pain impulses in the nervous system to draw the brain's attention to its loss. The brain could hardly fail to notice. Moreover, the very quality by which pain draws attention to itself – it is a form of sensory input that is hard to ignore – becomes a major burden when action has to be taken. Severe pain will hamper efforts to remedy matters – either by escaping or attending to the damage. The body needs some system for temporarily turning off the pain messages, and endorphins could be that system. By producing these chemicals the body is doing precisely what the doctors do when they administer morphine: activating the opiate receptors.

There is no disputing that the body has a system of some kind for modulating pain. The classic example is of men injured in battle who say, time and again, that even the most mutilating wounds provoked little pain or discomfort at the time they were inflicted, and sometimes for many hours afterwards. The evidence that endorphins are the answer is not conclusive, but very persuasive. One researcher, for example, found that injections of an endorphin could relieve the pain of patients with terminal cancer. And several studies have shown that non-pharmacological techniques of controlling pain, including electrical stimulation of nerves and acupuncture, can provoke the release of endorphins.

Placebo analgesia

In the late 1970s, Jon Levine, Newton Gordon and Howard Fields of the University of California were struck by the parallels between narcotic analgesia and placebo analgesia. Both tend to become less effective when used repeatedly over long periods; users of both methods may show a compulsion to keep taking them and to increase the dose; and both can evoke certain physiological changes (the abstinence syndrome) when users are denied them. The three Americans set out to examine the possible role of endorphins in placebo analgesia by designing experiments involving naloxone, the opiate antagonist drug.

Fifty or so volunteer patients were admitted to hospital for the surgical removal, under local anaesthetic, of impacted wisdom teeth. As a local anaesthetic wears off, patients experience a steadily increasing level of pain. Volunteers who had agreed to take part were told that two hours after the operation, when it would be normal to receive a pain-killer, they'd get one of the following three things: a dose of morphine; a dummy tablet; or a drug (naloxone) that might make the pain slightly worse. An hour later they'd receive another dose – again drawn at random from the agents on offer. They were also told that neither they nor the staff administering the drug would know (at the time of administration) who was getting what. At hourly intervals throughout the experiment the patients rated the amount of pain they were suffering.

The experimenters were interested only in those patients who had happened to receive a placebo on both occasions; a placebo on the first occasion followed by naloxone on the second occasion; or naloxone followed by placebo. The first thing that became clear was that patients who had received a placebo followed by naloxone experienced more pain than others who received two placebos. Naloxone was, as expected, making the pain worse.

Levine, Gordon and Fields then isolated subjects whose first drug had been a placebo, and compared those who *had* and *had not* responded to it. They defined responders as people whose pain rating remained constant or decreased one hour after receiving a placebo. Anyone whose pain went on increasing after being given a placebo was defined as a non-responder. The researchers next looked at the effects of a dose of naloxone on these two groups. They found that naloxone boosted the pain ratings of the placebo responders, such that their pain ended up equalling that of the non-responders.

The interpretation of these findings isn't easy, but it appears that placebo-induced pain relief is abolished by naloxone. Naloxone is known to counteract morphine-induced pain relief by displacing the morphine molecules from the opiate receptors. It is thus reasonable to conclude that when naloxone abolishes placebo-induced pain relief, it too does so by displacing endorphins from the receptors. In this case, then, the placebos worked by prompting the brain to instruct the body to increase its output of endorphins.

Pain, of course, is only one of many states and illnesses that can be mitigated by placebos. So there is little reason to suppose that *all* placebo effects are mediated by endorphins. Indeed, given the complexity and subtlety of living organisms, it would be rather surprising if there was only one mechanism. So what other biochemical or nervous interactions might also mediate the placebo effect?

Mind on body

Before considering other possible mechanisms, it would be as well to recall the great variety of circumstances in which there is now reasonably convincing evidence of physical health being swayed by states of mind.

The idea itself is far from new; one recent reviewer quotes

from an 1884 edition of the *British Medical Journal* on the subject of funerals: '... the depression of spirits under which the chief mourners labour on these occasions peculiarly predisposes them to some of the worst effects of chill'. For much of the past century, though, the notion that the mind has any very direct bearing on physical health has held greater sway among lay people than among doctors. The poet W. H. Auden has captured the belief perfectly in his ballad of 'Miss Gee', the tale of a lonely spinster who develops cancer. Later on the day of her diagnosis, her doctor, gloomily speculating on the nature of his patient's illness, likens cancer to a hidden assassin waiting to strike:

> 'Childless women get it,
> And men when they retire;
> It's as if there had to be some outlet
> For their foiled creative fire.'

The past couple of decades have witnessed a limited rediscovery of the effects of the mind on the body. The death of a spouse, for example, is reported to bring about a sharp increase in mortality among widowers, and a marked decline in the health of widows. On a rather different tack, chronic stress has also been held responsible for trench mouth in which normally harmless bacteria living on the gums and around the teeth turn pathogenic and cause severe inflammation and ulceration.

Staying with infection, a study carried out by Yale University at the end of the 1970s explored the psychosocial risk factors that predispose people to developing glandular fever. This illness is caused by an organism called the Epstein-Barr (EB) virus. Although it is pretty well ubiquitous, not everyone succumbs to it. Why? The Yale researchers devised a detailed survey of 1,400 cadets at West Point Military Academy. They first tested each cadet's blood for antibodies to the EB virus – the presence of such antibodies indicating that the individual concerned had already had the infection. This ruled out some two-thirds of the cadets; of the remainder, about a quarter developed clinical or sub-clinical glandular fever during the next four years. The aim of the researchers was to find a pattern that would distinguish those who did succumb to the EB virus from those who didn't. They used academic, psychosocial and other data about the students and their home backgrounds.

When all the findings were in, the analysis showed that the students most likely to develop glandular fever were the sons of fathers who were 'over-achievers' (in other words had an occupation with a status higher than might have been expected of their education or background); those with a strong commitment to a military career; those with a deeply-felt respect for certain aspects of a military life; and those who had scored poorly on their academic work. What all these individuals had in common was, presumably, a feeling of being under pressure; the implication is that this manifested itself in a reduced resistance to disease.

A very different kind of study on the way that life events affect health has come from McMaster University in Canada. In this case the researchers collected data on absenteeism from work among a group of steel workers before and after they were screened for high blood pressure. Those whose blood pressure was above a certain level were told that they were suffering from hypertension, the technical term for this condition. Thereafter, those so labelled began to take more days off work. One interpretation might, of course, have been that these individuals were genuinely more often sick. But this wouldn't explain why the absenteeism rose only after they'd been given their diagnosis. It might also have been a consequence of the treatment they had been given – except that absenteeism went up even in those who had not been prescribed any treatment. If the steel workers were not malingering – and the researchers do not seem to think they were – the only explanation was that being labelled 'hypertensive' had had a deleterious effect on their health. It had, to use the jargon term, encouraged them to adopt the 'sick role'.

Very different again is an ingenious and imaginative study by

Roger Ulrich, a geographer at the University of Delaware. His subjects were people admitted to hospital to have their gallstones removed, an operation that is normally followed by a week to ten days as an in-patient. The two-bedded wards in which all subjects spent this recovery period were identical in every respect save one: the view through the window. Some rooms faced on to a clump of deciduous trees, others on to a blank brick wall. Using the hospital records, which included the number of the room assigned to each patient, Ulrich was able to come up with twenty-three matched pairs of patients, half of whom had had a room with a view, and half of whom hadn't. He then compared their post-operative recovery.

The differences were striking. Patients with the better view required fewer pain-killing drugs and were able to leave hospital earlier.

Cancer and the mind

The disease that has received the most attention in respect of the mind is cancer. To demonstrate that certain states of mind predispose one to cancer is extremely difficult, and some of the studies that have been done contradict each other. But one of the best has used the Minnesota Multiphasic Personality Inventory (MMPI). This is a standard research method of assessing peoples' outlook and state of mind. More than 2000 employees of one American car firm who completed the MMPI were followed up for seventeen years. Slightly under a fifth of them were rated by this system as 'depressive'. In the long run they were almost twice as likely to develop cancer as non-depressed individuals.

In Britain, the psychiatrist Dr Stephen Greer has organized a series of studies on the psychological correlates of breast cancer. One of his analyses concerned women with a breast lump who were attending hospital for a biopsy. He showed that women whose lumps turned out to be malignant were of a type who, like Miss Gee in Auden's poem, rarely expressed any of the anger they felt. Greer and his colleagues also followed up women who'd been treated for breast cancer. They found that early death was associated with feelings of hopelessness; survival, on the other hand, was associated with fighting spirit or with a straightforward denial that the cancer was a problem.

Fascinating as it is to learn how non-material factors can influence the progress of an illness, the real pay-off from the patient's viewpoint would be some way of exploiting this understanding. Here too it is cancer that points the way. All sorts of approaches have been used from meditation to visualization – the latter being an attempt to mobilize the body's own defences by having patients imagine their tumour coming under attack. They're told to visualize this in whatever way they find easiest, some favouring biologically accurate images of white blood cells engulfing cancerous cells, others preferring to imagine the struggle in some other terms. But satisfying as patients may find this form of treatment, the evidence that it has any effect is still less than watertight.

By far the strongest evidence so far on the significance of non-material factors comes from David Spiegal and his co-workers at Stanford University in California. They wanted to find out if group therapy would have any effect on the survival of women with breast cancer. Of the eighty or so who agreed to take part, half received normal treatment, while half took part in group therapy sessions. The ninety-minute sessions were held at weekly intervals for a year. A psychiatrist or a social worker ran the groups, and the subjects discussed included how to cope with cancer, what it was like to have the disease, and the side effects of treatment. Patients learned how to use their experiences to help others, and some were taught a simple method of self-hypnosis to aid in pain control. The researchers followed up the women in the study for the next ten years. They found that those who had had therapy were living, on average, twice as long as those in the untreated group: a dramatic finding.

Why and how do these things happen? What is the nature of the link between a non-material influence – positive, such as group therapy for breast cancer, or negative, such as the effects of bereavement – and subsequent events? Several plausible mechanisms can be found by considering the impact that influences of this kind have on the immune system: on the arrangements by which the body deals with poisons, attack from microorganisms, and dead or abnormal cells.

Immune responses

The immune defence system is immensely complicated, but many of its actions depend on just three types of white blood cell. Macrophages can be found throughout the blood system and among the tissues. They act as scavengers of foreign or other unwanted material, and also co-operate with the other two cell types, called lymphocytes, in producing specific immunity. This is the process by which the body recognizes that hitherto unknown materials – the molecules coating the outside of a bacterium, for example – are foreign, attacks them, and then develops a more or less permanent memory of their precise nature. The next time these materials appear in the body they will be recognized for what they are. And the attack will be quicker, more vigorous, and quite specific in its target.

Some of the experimental work designed to demonstrate that psychological factors can affect the immune system has been carried out on animals. One popular test of immune function is to remove some of the animal's lymphocytes, place them in a test tube, and stimulate them with a chemical that is known to encourage them to proliferate. The faster their numbers multiply, the more effective is the animal's immune system thought to be functioning. A number of experiments have shown that if animals are subjected to stress of various kinds – the fear of receiving an electric shock, for example – their lymphocyte function becomes suppressed. Likewise, lymphocyte functioning is abnormally low in monkeys that have suffered maternal separation during the first year of life. The pattern that emerges from these and other such experiments is that acute and stimulating stress tends to give the immune system a boost, while chronic stress and frustration depress it.

Stress mechanisms

A variety of experiments of this kind have also been organized using humans. Typical was one carried out at a dental school in Boston, Massachusetts. The subjects were first-year students who agreed to submit themselves to various physiological and psychological measures that would be made on five occasions over the course of one academic year. Three of the selected dates coincided with important examinations; the other two were in more relaxed periods. The tests themselves comprised a questionnaire designed to measure the students' perceived levels of stress, and an assay of the amount of one type of antibody in their saliva – antibodies being the blood proteins that stick to foreign material and accelerate its destruction. The findings showed that the production of antibodies was lowest during periods of high stress – and, by implication, that the immune defences were at their weakest during this time.

Other work of this kind has featured all sorts of people and social groups. Loneliness in a group of psychiatric patients has been associated with a weakened immune response; so have bereavement, unemployment and marriage breakdown. Clinical depression is a condition in which you might expect to find the immune system working below par; indeed, it is a further part of folk wisdom that you're more susceptible to disease when you're feeling below par. Several studies have, in fact, shown that various elements of the immune response seem to function less well in people with depression.

There are, most likely, a whole raft of mechanisms by which these disparate events and states of mind can influence the workings of the immune system. Nothing in this field is certain. Much attention has been focused on a material called cortisol, sometimes referred to as stress hormone. The sequence of events leading to its release could go something like this. When stressed, the brain instructs a small part of its structure called the hypothalamus to produce a local hormone, corticotropin releasing factor. This stimulates the adjacent pituitary gland to secrete another hormone called ACTH, short for adrenocorticotrophic hormone. As its mouthful of a name implies, once ACTH has been released into the bloodstream it reaches, among other places, the outer layer or cortex of the adrenal glands, adjacent to the kidneys. These are the glands that actually secrete cortisol, the steroid hormone that affects the cells taking part in the immune response.

Cortisol may not be the only hormone to play a part in these matters. And neurotransmitters could also be involved in modulating the activity of the immune system. When a message travels through the body from one place to another, it passes along a chain of nerve cells, each separated from its neighbour by a narrow gap. The arrival of the nerve impulse at one of these gaps causes the membrane at that point to release a tiny quantity of a particular chemical. This diffuses across the gap and, when it reaches the membrane of the adjacent nerve, triggers another impulse, so ensuring that the message is relayed on down the next nerve. A number of experiments, in test tubes and in live animals, have shown that immune cells respond to these neurotransmitter chemicals.

Besides these chemical influences of the brain over the workings of the immune defence system, there is evidence of more direct control via the nervous system. The attempt to unravel these various influences has led to the creation of a new science with the descriptive but unwieldy title of psychoneuroimmunology. It seems destined to have a lively and interesting future.

Ubiquitous stress

'Stress' has become, in the past couple of decades, one of the most overworked words in the English language. So before passing on, it may be worth considering what it actually means. The difficulty arises because different people use it to mean different things. Anything unpleasant for which there is no immediately available remedy is apt to be labelled 'stressful'. The faintly clinical connotations of the word give an added importance to what might sound trivial if described merely as 'worrying' or 'upsetting'. Like any such catch-all concept it can be useful. Noisy neighbours, travelling in the rush hour, working on a factory production line, getting a divorce, moving house, preparing for an examination, and looking after an elderly and demented relative may all be described as stressful. When a word can be used so often and in so many unrelated circumstances, it is on the way towards meaning nothing at all.

Evolution, of course, has endowed humans with the ability to face difficult circumstances. The realization that the fire lit to deter animal intruders has gone out, and that a wolf is even now snuffling around the fringes of the camp, prompts the brain to effect a series of changes in body chemistry and physiology that prepare it to do one of two things: fight off the wolf; or, if it looks exceptionally intimidating, flee with all speed up the nearest tree. The 'fight or flight' response is a shorthand description for a whole set of bodily changes provoked by circumstances in which survival depends on either doing battle with a particular threat, or escaping it. It begins when the brain, via the nervous system, instructs several of the body's organ systems to undertake a series of actions that are then reinforced by an outpouring of certain hormones, notably adrenalin. This flurry of nervous and chemical messages causes blood to be diverted from the bowel and stomach to the muscles. Digestion, in other words, is put on hold and the more immediate business of fighting or fleeing takes priority in the competition for oxygen and nutrients.

A few of the hazards of modern city life are much as they ever were: in confrontations with a gang of youths in search of a wallet to steal, the 'fight or flight' response is as useful as ever. But much of the stress faced by urban dwellers is chronic (the factory production line) and unavoidable (travelling in the rush hour). These experiences prompt anger or distress or some other such emotion, and each will provoke some degree of arousal. But if there is nothing then and there to be done, this physiological arousal serves no purpose; it only exacerbates the discomfort. What were once a set of useful bodily responses have become, at best, mentally and physically irrelevant and at worst damaging, including to the operation of the immune system.

What all this has revealed is that many sorts of non-material influence can affect the body for good or ill. And these different influences almost certainly operate through more than one and maybe even dozens of different mechanisms.

Stress and the placebo effect

For several reasons, this understanding is relevant to the placebo effect. It seems highly likely that some at least of the mechanisms by which stress damages health are simply the reverse of those by which the placebo effect restores it. Most people spend most of their lives in an emotional middle range: neither sunk in gloom, nor raised to ecstasy. When these more extreme states of mind do impinge, they evoke responses that, positive or negative, have corresponding effects on the well-being of the person experiencing them.

Most important, this survey of non-material influences on health illustrates how the concept of the placebo effect is simply a rather specific variant of a phenomenon that is universal in human existence: that the impact of our lives and our surroundings on our state of mind has a bearing on our physical as well as our mental well-being. It is a reflection of the human fascination with misery and disaster that most of the studies that have been done concentrate on adverse influences. But though they're relatively thin on the ground, attempts have also been made to show that desirable circumstances or events have an enhancing effect on health. Pet ownership reduces the death rate among people who've suffered a heart attack; social support of all kinds diminishes the adverse effects of disaster; just the act of stroking a dog can lower the blood pressure!

A doctor who prescribes a pharmacologically ineffective but much desired tonic to one of his or her patients will be regarded as giving a placebo, and thereby exercising a medical function. If he or she smiles at the patients when they come into the surgery, shakes hands, and pays sympathetic attention to what they have to say, he or she will be applauded for politeness, but not considered as having done anything of particular medical significance. If the patient, on reaching home, gets an unexpected phone call from a loved and much-missed son or daughter asking to visit, we'll rejoice in that person's happiness, but probably won't think of it as having much to do with health. The facts presented in this chapter suggest that all three of these events are, in fact, qualitatively similar. What alternative or complementary medicine has achieved is to recognize, consciously or otherwise, that influences on health do not stop at the door of the consulting room, and that there are more ways of affecting health than doing physical things to the body. It is for this reason that orthodox medicine has something to learn from the activities of alternative practitioners, including – or perhaps especially – those whose philosophy and treatments seem utterly remote from the cool rationality of medical science.

PART TWO: Two Styles of Medicine

4 Into the Consulting Rooms

Differences in the practice of orthodox and complementary medicine

Virtually all of us have had first-hand experience of orthodox medicine, and a growing number have made at least one or two visits to a complementary practitioner of some kind. The brief case histories that follow will serve to underline some of the key differences between orthodox and complementary medicine, especially the ways in which these two enterprises go about their business. Each account is based largely on fact, albeit a blend of more than one patient with more than one practitioner. There is nothing exceptional about the conditions or the consultations; thousands of patients with comparable problems meet thousands of practitioners every day. First, then, the orthodox approach.

Orthodox medicine: case 1

Bill, a man in his early forties, began to experience bouts of pain and stiffness in his right knee. From time to time it would seize up while he was sitting working or watching television. Straightening it then caused him pain – as did going downstairs, though not up. Not someone inclined to visit the doctor more often than he needed, Bill ignored the problem for as long as he could. But at the back of his mind there was one worry; that this might be the first hint of arthritis.

Eventually he did visit the doctor. Although he'd been

registered with his GP for ten years, neither Bill nor the doctor could claim to know one another. The consultation, conducted at the usual brisk pace, lasted between four and five minutes. The GP made a cursory examination of the appearance and feel of the knee. He asked Bill to flex and extend it twice, and said he could detect a faint creaking. He suggested that Bill had probably banged it, and that the symptoms were no more than a late indication of damage that was now healing. However, he told Bill to arrange for an X-ray at the local teaching hospital and in the meantime he prescribed pain-killing drugs. These were quite effective.

Arranging for the X-ray took about a fortnight, and it was a further five days before the results were phoned through to the GP. There was nothing to see on the X-ray, and the GP referred Bill to the orthopaedic outpatient clinic at the local hospital. This took another three weeks. Although Bill had the first appointment of the afternoon, the consultant who was to examine him arrived thirty minutes late. After a further fifteen minutes – while Bill waited, minus his trousers, in a cubicle – the consultant entered, examined the knee, felt its movement, confirmed that the X-ray showed no signs of arthritis, and added his opinion that the symptoms were most likely a consequence of some forgotten injury. Throughout this short consultation the doctor remained, if not uninterested, then wholly detached. Having told Bill to come back if the problem didn't clear up of its own accord, he left. Fortunately, the problem did clear up. Bill's only recollection of the consultant as a person was that he'd been wearing his white coat with the collar turned up. Bill couldn't decide if this was an oversight or some curious affectation.

Orthodox medicine: case 2

Joe was in his early thirties when, washing himself in the bath one evening, he discovered a lump on the side of his right testicle. Although not given to assuming that each lump beneath

INTO THE CONSULTING ROOMS

the skin is malignant, the word 'cancer' came to Joe's mind. The GP, a brusque woman, confirmed the existence of the lump, and said she didn't know what had caused it. Joe raised the possibility that it might be malignant, but the GP – whether or not she realized how concerned Joe was – made little attempt to offer comfort or reassurance. She fixed an NHS appointment for Joe at the local hospital – but there was a three-week wait. Within a couple of days Joe had convinced himself that the worst had happened and found the prospect of waiting three weeks unbearable. He cancelled the NHS appointment and made another to see the same consultant privately.

This consultation took place within three days and lasted more than twenty minutes. The doctor's opinion was that the lump was benign, but that the possibility of something worse couldn't be entirely ruled out until some rather elaborate radiological investigations had been done. These were arranged for the following week. Joe was required to spend the better part of an hour on the table of an X-ray room while radio-opaque dyes were injected into various parts of his body. As a scientist, Joe has a greater than average grasp of biology and medicine; but it wasn't clear to him what the investigations might reveal. The radiologist in charge was not helpful, and suggested that Joe should ask the consultant who had originally requested the investigations. Joe had, in fact, done this but, as is often the case, the stress of the consultation had prevented him from fully grasping what was to be done and why. In the event, the tests were negative and in due course the lumps receded of their own accord.

Were these examples of good medicine or bad? Neither Bill nor Joe were inclined to complain about the treatment they had received. They had gone to their doctors with specific symptoms, which had been investigated and found not to pose a threat. They had had the benefit of specialist opinions from acknowledged experts. On one level it was all very satisfactory; but on another it was not.

There had been little time for talking, for putting them at their ease; even the private consultation had been relatively impersonal. You'd expect more of an attempt than this to establish a relationship when taking the car for a service. In fairness to doctors, they too would prefer a more leisurely pace of activity – such as can indeed be supplied outside the public sector. And it would, of course, be unfair to generalize from these consultations to the millions that take place every year. Many NHS doctors do make conscious efforts to treat their patients as people. Some have devoted considerable thought to the matter. Dr David Mendel, lately of St Thomas's Hospital in London, is the author of a book entitled *Proper Doctoring*. This has a whole section devoted to the relationship between doctors and patients: how to foster it, and why it may go wrong. His thoughts on reassurance in medicine are the conclusions of a humane man looking back on a lifetime in medicine. He writes:

Most people who consult doctors have no 'disease' other than the ageing process, or the symptoms of abuse of their physique. Many other patients have overestimated the implications of their symptoms, so reassurance is one of the main therapeutic weapons, and it may well be the most important. When you have done a particularly good job in reassurance, patients often say, 'Well, I'm sorry to have wasted your time, doctor.' I tell them that far from wasting my time, my favourite medicine is soundly-based reassurance ... Train yourself to derive more satisfaction from reassuring patients than giving them drugs. Unlike so many drugs, it actually does the patients good.

Technology figured in both Bill and Joe's stories; and whenever technology enters the picture it tends to dominate the action. The radiological investigation that featured in Bill's second hospital appointment is hardly state of the art technology; yet on this occasion, and despite his residual fears about his condition, Bill might as well have been a piece of machinery brought into the factory for a routine service. The staff operating such equipment are not indifferent to the people on the receiving end of their investigations. But the instruments absorb most of their attention; there's little left over for the patient.

In all cases, the questions put to the patients by their doctors – GPs and consultants – were closely confined to the immediate problem. They made no attempt to enquire about the patients' more general health and well-being, or what they were thinking or feeling. They made no attempt to discover if either patient was distressed by his illness – which Joe certainly was. Nor were Joe's worries tackled when he made it clear to both his doctors that he was seriously scared by the prospect that he might have a malignant tumour. We shall turn now to complementary medicine.

Complementary medicine: case 1

Joan, in her early thirties, had two problems: the inside of her right foot was giving her pain, and she felt tension and stiffness in her neck. The practitioner she chose to visit used acupuncture, manipulation and various homeopathic remedies. He looked on himself as a practitioner of natural medicine. Joan went to see him because conventional doctoring had failed to eliminate the pain in her foot, and she had had previous good experiences with complementary medicine.

The practitioner decided to begin with Joan's foot. Joan explained that the problem had started after some strenuous walking; the foot had swollen up and now, several months on, the pain was recurring each time she played tennis, or walked on rough ground. The physiotherapist at the local hospital had talked of her Achilles tendon being rather tight, and recommended some exercises. But these hadn't done the trick.

The practitioner then asked Joan if she had experienced pain anywhere else in her body. Apart from her neck, a problem that predated the foot injury, Joan told him that she had had some pain in her lower back. He also asked a series of questions about her general health, and the past illnesses or injuries she'd had, particularly those involving sprains or strains. He also wanted to know about Joan's job (office work), and about her appetite, diet and eating habits.

About ten minutes into the consultation he asked her to lie on a couch so that he could begin his physical examination. He first took her pulse. He examined her feet, feeling each closely, and comparing the injured one with its counterpart. He noticed that the feet were distinctly different in size, explained more or less in passing how this had come about (one arch was more prominent than the other) and what she could do about it. By manipulating each joint of the foot, and palpating the soft tissues in search of tender points, he tracked down the source of the problem.

His conclusion was that Joan had probably strained some of the ligaments supporting the arch of her foot. He suggested four remedies. First, he gave her ten to fifteen minutes of massage. To further stimulate the flow of blood to the local tissues, he used acupuncture: half a dozen needles in various parts of the affected foot, and one more needle slightly higher up in each leg. These were left in place for fifteen to twenty minutes. The other two treatments were for Joan herself to do at home. One was hydrotherapy; Joan had to soak her foot regularly for fifteen minutes in a bowl of hot water containing a tablespoon of Epsom salts. He also told her to rub it with a cream containing the homeopathic remedy ruta, and to apply a cold compress before going to bed.

Joan's history of strains and sprains suggested that her ligaments and tendons were not as strong as they might have been. In the longer term he thought that some changes in diet might do something to improve matters.

The consultation had already lasted over forty minutes, and the next patient was waiting. The practitioner removed the acupuncture needles, and suggested that Joan made another appointment to deal with the neck problems.

A week later she returned. The foot problem had not gone, but was giving her less trouble. The practitioner examined her neck. He felt the muscles of her neck and shoulder and declared them to be unduly tense. With Joan sitting on the couch he asked her to rotate her neck slowly from left to right, while holding it in his hands. Following further gentle manipulation of the bones in her neck he concluded that one of the two main vertebrae were out of alignment. To overcome this he turned Joan round, clasped her neck and one arm in what resembled a wrestling move, and applied a quick thrust. The neck bones responded with an audible crack. He followed this with ten minutes of massage. The consultation – just under thirty minutes – finished with some advice on diet, and a brief discussion of the value of vitamin supplements.

Complementary medicine: case 2

Mavis, in her late fifties and a bit of a worrier, was going through an even more worrying time than usual. She'd been diagnosed as having an hiatus hernia, and the hospital consultant had told her that he wanted to perform an endoscopy. Mavis knew what was involved because a relative had undergone the same procedure a year or two previously. She spent a week getting herself psyched up to face the ordeal – only to receive a last minute phone call postponing the appointment for ten days. This proved to be the last straw; she became acutely anxious; she began sleeping badly. So she went to see the herbalist she had consulted the last time her nerves had become troublesome. Her GP had already offered her Valium; but Mavis had read a lot about the risks of addiction to minor tranquillizers. She felt safer taking a herbal remedy – particularly as the one she had taken previously had been so effective.

Although the herbalist grasped the nature of the problem within a couple of minutes, and looked in her notes to see what she had taken last time, he didn't go immediately to the dispensary. Instead he asked Mavis to tell him about her health since he had last seen her, and about the events that had led to the hospital appointment. He was not aiming to intrude on territory being explored by the hospital, but he wanted to get a full picture.

He didn't press Mavis for detail, but with his open, enquiring and sympathetic manner he didn't need to. Ten minutes into the consultation Mavis became much calmer, and explained the difficulties she'd been having in swallowing. The herbalist suggested she try some slippery elm. This can be made into a nourishing gruel that is easy to swallow. Mavis also mentioned that she had developed an ache in the base of her neck that had spread to her shoulders. The practitioner examined the area, felt it, and suggested that it was most likely to be another consequence of the stress she had been suffering. He recommended some exercises that involved pulling the shoulders back, rotating the head and breathing deeply.

For Mavis's anxiety and insomnia the herbalist prescribed a mixture of valerian, skullcap and motherwort. But what might, in a different context, have been a call to pick up a repeat prescription had instead become a complete health check that lasted almost thirty minutes.

In almost every respect these two consultations were quite unlike those with the orthodox practitioners. They were long, they purposely covered territory seemingly remote from the problems that had prompted them; and the patients, far from feeling that the consultations had been incomplete, were extremely satisfied. In these cases, describing the interaction between patient and practitioner as a relationship is appropriate. When consultations take only four minutes, most of which is spent scribbling case-notes or writing on the prescription pad, the word 'relationship' seems quite hollow. So is this a better form of medicine than the examples from orthodox medicine seem to suggest?

It could be argued that while every NHS GP would like to spend thirty minutes with his or her patients, it just isn't feasible. A more aggressive response might be that a great deal of what passed between patients and practitioners was, at best, mere pleasantry and, at worst, wastefully irrelevant to solving the problems that had prompted the patients to seek help.

Two perspectives, then; and two opposed views of what medicine is for, and how best to please patients.

5 A Crooked Path
A brief history of orthodox medicine

In just a few generations we have come to expect results from medicine that would have been unimaginable to anyone born before the beginning of this century. This success has flowed from the application of science. But it was a long time coming – which is why, as pointed out in Chapter 2, the history of medicine's limited achievements prior to the nineteenth century is to a great extent the history of reliance on the placebo effect.

Medicine of some sort or another must be almost as old as our species itself. From the time that humans first developed self-awareness, and first showed the kind of consciousness characteristic of *Homo sapiens*, they must have been thinking of ways in which to improve their lives. The development of medicine has been a long and faltering process of detachment from spiritual and supernatural explanations of disease, and a slow acceptance of largely materialist explanations. In this respect the history of medicine has paralleled the history of science, and indeed the wider history of most Western societies.

For obvious reasons there are no written records of our distant ancestors' first tentative attempts at overcoming disease or coping with injury. The closest we can come to an understanding of what they might have achieved is through studying the medicine of the few remaining primitive cultures of which we have direct experience: the Amerindians, for example, or the Australian Aborigines. Medicine at this stage of human development was inseparable from religion and from magic.

Individuals and communities needed some way of making sense of the periodic plagues and pestilences against which they had so little defence; how else to explain them except by invoking some kind of divine being seeking to express his anger? And how else to console themselves that something could be done than by casting spells, making sacrifices and mixing magic potions?

Common experience, though, would have taught our ancestors of the benefits of warmth and cold in alleviating symptoms. Primitive peoples have invariably made use of extracts of herbs, roots and other plant materials – some at least of which would have had a real and perhaps even beneficial pharmacological effect. More formal systems of medicine came later. Certainly there seem to have been full-time physicians of some kind in Mesopotamia.

Egyptian medicine made little advance beyond that of the Babylonians, and major developments had to await the Greeks. Hippocrates and his followers left many written works, and we know much about his views on the nature of health and disease. He observed and recorded individual cases in great detail, and tried to relate disease to the climate and other features of the environment. Although often wrong, he was setting about the business of medicine in a way that would be recognizable to today's doctors.

First ethics

In one sphere in particular his name as well as his influence remains strong: the ethics of medical practice as represented by the famous Hippocratic Oath. 'I will not use my position to indulge in sexual contacts with the bodies of women or of men ... Whatever I hear, professionally or privately, which ought not to be divulged, I will keep secret and tell no one.' These and other passages are little different from the codes of ethics under which today's doctors still practise.

Another passage instructs the physician not to cut, even for the removal of bladder stones: in other words, not to perform surgery. '... I will leave such procedures to the practitioners of that craft'. The separation between medicine and surgery, and the slight disdain with which those who exercise the latter skill are still viewed by those practising the former dates from this time. And this, of course, casts a more self-serving light on the Oath. Parts of it are really a code of restrictive practices designed to keep those not of the fraternity out of the healing business. 'I will hand on precepts, lectures and all other learning to my sons, to those of my master and pupils duly apprenticed and sworn, and to none other.' There is a strong whiff here of the closed shop that foreshadows the disputes between orthodox medicine and its competitors that have continued up to the present. Today's hostility is one further manifestation of an antagonism that has always existed.

This, of course, raises the question of what we mean by 'orthodox' medicine. The boundaries today are more straightforward than they were in former times because 'orthodox' has become more or less synonymous with 'scientific'. These boundaries are not immutable; indeed, the whole point of science is that its methods are subversive. After some pushing and shoving a more powerful truth will displace a weaker one. But even though the boundaries may move, it's not usually too difficult to say what lies within them at any one time. The orthodoxies of previous times were not so easily delineated. There was no universally accepted theory by which to define orthodoxy. Under such circumstances an orthodox system of medicine can be identified only in terms of its usage and approval by the majority, or by what we would now refer to as the 'establishment'. As often as not, orthodoxy was what those with religious or political power said it was. No further justification was necessary – or, indeed, available.

The other great name in Greek medicine is, of course, Aristotle. He did much to establish the view of disease as shaped by four humours and four qualities. The humours were blood, phlegm, black bile and white bile; the qualities were hot, dry, wet and cold. Illness could be thought of as a disturbance of the relative proportions of these elements in the body. Although without foundation, this essentially poetic view of health and disease was sufficiently appealing to remain the basis of much medical explanation for the next two millenia.

The Romans to the Renaissance

With the rise of the Roman Empire, the Greek tradition of medicine established itself throughout Europe. Despite the dynamism of the Empire in military matters, trade and colonial administration, medicine advanced little during its half-millennium sway. The one man from this era whose reputation did soar, and remained high for centuries, was Galen. Although his theories of medicine and physiology were treated for centuries almost as holy writ, they were entirely wrong. They comprised claims about the importance and nature of a mishmash of fluids with names like 'natural spirit' and 'vital spirit' that were presumed to ebb and flow around the body.

In Europe the Middle Ages were an even less interesting period for medicine. While considerable advances were made in Chinese and Arabic medicine, in Christian countries the dead hand of the powerful and dogmatic Church inhibited original and challenging thought about the natural world. Medically speaking, it was not a good time to be alive.

From the viewpoint of the patient, the Renaissance was not a great deal better. But the more thoughtful would at least have had the consolation of living in an age when attempts to advance knowledge once again prospered. Copernicus challenged the view that the Earth lay at the centre of the Universe by claiming that the Sun occupied that position. Medicine found its own Copernicus in Paracelsus, the Swiss physician who became professor of medicine at Basel in 1527. He publicly burnt the works of Galen, thereby offering one of the first hints that, just as astronomy had begun to rid itself of dogma and start matching its view of the world to observational data, so too should medicine.

The intellectual cobwebs having, as it were, been shaken out, the pace of change in medicine began slowly to accelerate. The Renaissance saw the beginnings of professionalism as physicians, apothecaries, midwives and barber-surgeons began to set up systems of entry into their occupations, with training and even examinations.

Medicine advances

The pace quickened further in the seventeenth century, the age of Galileo, Newton, Descartes and Boyle. A scientific world view began increasingly to influence medicine. The physician who dominated English medicine during this period was William Harvey. At that time, blood was still thought to ebb and flow within the body. Harvey's classic observations on the role of the valves within veins demonstrated that they allow blood to flow only in one direction: towards the heart. Technology, too, played an important role in this era. This was the century in which the microscope became available to medical researchers.

One major development in philosophy during the seventeenth century reverberates even now. It was the theory of dualism put forward by the French philosopher René Descartes in his book *Discourse on Method*. Arguing the separateness of body and mind, he declared that the former was made up of substance, which has length, breadth and depth and can be measured and divided; the latter, the 'thinking substance', has none of these physical properties and is indivisible. The brain and the rest of the central nervous system are in the first category; the thoughts, desires, emotions and the rest of the activity which goes on inside them are in the second. Although Cartesian dualism, as it became known, was a stimulus to the development of objective science and the scientific method, it also contributed to the relatively tardy development of the science and medicine of the mind.

A CROOKED PATH

The eighteenth century saw more in the way of consolidation than major advance. Surgery, however, moved ahead under the influence of the surgeon John Hunter. His determination to improve on existing operations and to develop new ones led him to animal experiments – and helped to lay the foundations for a more scientific approach to what had hitherto been a craft.

One other name from this period remains familiar even to people outside medicine: a country doctor called Edward Jenner. Jenner inoculated people with cowpox, and showed that they then became immune to the more virulent smallpox. In truth it wasn't his own observations that inspired the action, and he wasn't the first individual to test the principle of what we now call immunisation. But he did set about it more systematically than others – no less, perhaps, than might be expected of a former pupil of the great John Hunter!

With the nineteenth century came the Industrial Revolution and the emergence of an urban working class plagued by poverty, overcrowding, poor nutrition, bad housing and all the rest of what we now describe as Dickensian conditions. Reformers were genuinely appalled by the way in which the poor of cities like London and Liverpool lived their lives. Their demands for change fostered what has been called the 'sanitary idea': the great schemes to develop proper sewerage and to bring clean drinking water to the areas of greatest squalor.

These developments took place against a backdrop of radically changing views of society. Karl Marx devised a new political philosophy: one complementary, at least in his own mind, to the equally radical ideas about the nature of man and the origins of species being developed by Charles Darwin. This was the age in which medicine established itself as an enterprise with its theoretical underpinnings – if not always its practice – firmly rooted in science. Specialization too began to feature in medicine.

The germ theory of disease

In respect of understanding, preventing, and eventually treating disease, the highlight of the nineteenth century was the advent of the germ theory of disease. This swept away centuries of misconceptions about evil spirits, miasmas and scores of other factors believed to be responsible for a host of diseases. The man whose experimental ingenuity offered the all-important insight was Louis Pasteur. Another biologist, Robert Koch, discovered the bacterium responsible for one of the great killers, tuberculosis. He also spelt out a set of conditions, known as Koch's postulates, to be met before a given disorder can be reliably attributed to a specific microbe. The organism must, for example, be found in all cases of the disease, and be capable of causing this disease when isolated and injected into an animal. With this demonstration of the value of disciplined logic in trying to understand the natural world, the science of bacteriology was on its way.

The consequences of the germ theory of disease sometimes proved extremely unpopular. The case of Dr Semmelweiss in Vienna shows how even proof may not be enough to overcome prejudice. Working in an obstetric hospital, he was all too aware of the number of women dying of puerperal fever. By systematically checking, he found that the women most at risk were those being attended by doctors who had conducted or been present at autopsies carried out on other women with the disease. Although knowing nothing of bacteria, Semmelweiss rightly inferred that the problem might stem from something that had contaminated the doctors' hands, and he therefore suggested that they make a habit of washing before carrying out any examination. In spite of clear evidence that this simple manoeuvre reduced the death rate, Semmelweiss was ostracized for making such an audacious suggestion.

Surgery, too, was a beneficiary of the germ theory. Surgeons of that era paid no special attention to hygiene. To perform their bloody and brutal operations they wore old, already blood-spattered clothes. Patients who didn't bleed to death or die of a subsequent wound infection could count themselves lucky. Joseph Lister was one of the first doctors to realize that the best way of preventing wound infection is to keep live bacteria from entering in the first place. For this purpose he designed a piece of apparatus that sprayed the disinfectant carbolic acid into the air above and around the wound.

The more immediate horror of surgery lay in the operation itself – conducted without benefit of anaesthesia. Assistants were required to hold down the patients ('victims' would be a more appropriate word) while the surgeon sliced and sawed. Surgical reputations depended less on skill than on speed. But blessed relief began to dawn with the first use, in 1844, of nitrous oxide to remove a tooth.

At the beginning of this century, most of what doctors knew about their patients came from looking at them, feeling them, and asking questions. Then diagnostic instruments began to appear. The simplest, the stethoscope, was invented by Laennec as a single tube applied to just one ear. It was to become so widely used that it grew to symbolize medicine. In an altogether different league of diagnostic sophistication was Röntgen's discovery of X-rays.

The advent of professionalism

Hospitals themselves underwent a great improvement during the nineteenth century. When Florence Nightingale travelled to Scutari to nurse soldiers wounded in the Crimean War, she was disgusted by what she found. By sheer determination, and in the face of considerable indifference to the plight of the unfortunate men she was trying to help, she managed to improve their conditions. After the war, intent on training other women to follow her example, she chose St Thomas's Hospital in London as the home of the world's first school of nursing. Its foundation marked the advent of professionalism in nursing: an important reform of what had hitherto been a menial job undertaken by women of low status, and often after little or no training.

Professionalism was also on the increase among doctors. Entry continued to be controlled by the handful of largely self-serving Royal Colleges, but by the end of the century these bodies had begun to take their responsibilities – setting examinations and the like – more seriously. Even so, Parliament felt obliged to intervene. The result was the Medical Act of 1858. This set up the General Medical Council to maintain a register of properly qualified doctors, set standards of conduct, give guidance on the university curriculum, and inspect medical schools to ensure that their students were being properly educated.

With time the straightforward division into surgeons and physicians became progressively less able to cope with the growing body of knowledge. The scene was being set for the division and sub-division of specialities that is a feature of hospital medicine in the twentieth century.

With science providing its theoretical base and its research methodology, medical knowledge underwent a seemingly exponential growth. And whereas nineteenth century biologists and doctors were mainly concerned with the workings of whole organs, or sometimes the tissues of which they're made, their twentieth century counterparts have learnt to study these same functions at cellular and even molecular level.

After slow progress in the first part of the century, immunology grew rapidly. Once the mechanism of graft rejection had been understood, ways could be found to suppress it – and transplantation programmes designed to deal with failed kidneys, hearts, livers and other organs could be embarked on.

Science as the driving force

Gregor Mendel, working in the nineteenth century in the obscurity of a monastery in what is now Czechoslavakia, demonstrated the pattern by which the characteristics of an organism are inherited. In 1953, Francis Crick and James Watson

A CROOKED PATH

discovered how the make-up of the long molecules of DNA found in the nucleus of every cell in the body acts as code by which to store the information making up that inheritance. Within thirty years, biologists had learned not only how to read the code, but also how to manipulate it. Genetic engineering has made it possible, in principle, to overcome the adverse effects of bad or missing genes, and even to create completely new ones. Inherited disease no longer seems inescapable.

Pharmacology has yielded thousands of drugs for influencing virtually every aspect of body function. Asthmatics can now lead a relatively normal existence, untroubled by life-threatening constrictions of the airways; schizophrenics whose lives would once have been spent in an asylum can return to the community; and all manner of bacterial diseases are overcome using antibiotics.

In nearly all these enterprises, the key developments have depended as much on basic research as on attempts to solve particular problems. Many of the most valuable advances have come from scientists driven more by a wish to understand the body than to heal it. The speed with which researchers were able to work out the cause of AIDS and then to begin testing drugs and vaccines was the fruit of a generation of investigators who had studied the molecular biology of viruses in the same spirit as their predecessors had investigated the physiology of much larger organisms. Despite periodic claims to the contrary, all the evidence suggests that useful knowledge accrues most rapidly by backing the efforts of researchers with good ideas, even if their current relevance to human illness is uncertain.

Different rules, of course, apply in the development of new medical technologies; but the growth this century has been equally impressive. Non-invasive methods of treatment have been boosted by the invention of fibre-optics: flexible bundles of glass fibres that allow doctors to peer through the fine viewing tubes now available for insertion into almost every bodily orifice. Equally fine instruments can be used to remove a gallstone or snip out a growth in the colon without the need first to slice open the patient's body.

Not without faults

This hymn of praise for the achievements of medicine should not be taken to mean that it is without fault or limitation. Many advances in well-being have stemmed not from health care as such, but from better food, housing and the like. The emphasis on cure has left preventive and public health medicine in a state of relative neglect; technological enthusiasm has often run ahead of the sober assessments needed to decide if this or that gizmo or gadget really justifies its often horrendous cost. With all the 'simple' disease problems now solved, further progress demands ever greater resources – which is why the focus of world medical research shifted to the United States. The peaks yet to be conquered include the chronic degenerative disorders like arthritis; those conditions, such as heart disease, that appear to stem in large measure from the way we live; and, of course, the great unmentionable of this age, cancer. Overcoming these problems will continue to demand huge and continuing expenditure – and to what end? In the long run, as someone once said, we're all dead. How awful if the result of all this ingenuity was not to allow us to remain fit and healthy until the inevitable end, but merely to add extra years to a life lived out in decrepitude: spared death from this and that, but burdened with an existence lacking all quality.

As measured by falling death rates and rising longevity – though, for most of them, in few other ways – the major beneficiaries of modern medicine have been the poor in the Third World. But death control in the absence of birth control has too frequently outstripped the capacity of the people to develop the educational, social and agricultural arrangements that would have allowed their rising populations to enjoy a greater lifespan. Matters have reached crisis point; doctors whose whole lives have been devoted to public health in the tropics are questioning the wisdom and even the humanity of mass immunization and other campaigns that may prevent undernourished children dying of infectious disease, but instead condemn them to death by starvation as adults.

The negative public perception of modern medicine is an issue I'll return to in the next chapter. Some of the criticism is justified, much is not; but the weaknesses and contradictions shouldn't be allowed to disguise the fact that scientific medicine, as much as science itself, has proved to be an intellectual and practical triumph. Other forms of medicine may co-exist with it – Ayurvedic medicine in India, for example – but only scientific medicine is global.

Science and medicine

Medicine did not hitch itself to science at one time or in one place. But that's hardly surprising, because science itself did not come into existence at a particular moment. Observation is the first prerequisite of any kind of scientific understanding. The Greeks placed more store by thought and discussion, which correspondingly limited their chances of scientific progress. The emergence of Christianity as a powerful force gave it virtual control over all branches of learning for many hundreds of years. Religious men saw little virtue and some hazard in the questioning that underpins scientific enquiry. Medical progress in particular was inhibited by the Church's disapproval of dissection. Only with the Renaissance, with the escape from the stranglehold of the Church, was it again possible to adopt the sceptical, questioning attitudes on which science depends. Thereafter its progress was swift and triumphant.

To say that medicine has become scientific is not to imply that its progress has been linear or without blind alleys, misdirections and disasters. Science may be a system of intellectual navigation, but it doesn't offer a pre-drawn map. The researcher sketches the map as he progresses. From time to time he realizes that he has lost his way. At such moments it is necessary to erase as much of the map as it takes to return to a position of certainty, and then set out again. Such hopeful forays and tactical withdrawals are not a failure of science; they *are* science. The realization of error is painful for the investigator and, in the case of medical science, may prove even more calamitous for the unfortunate patient. But it is hard to see how, even with the greatest prudence, all such reversals might be avoided.

Could medicine have chosen not to attach itself to science, to this particular way of understanding the world? Clearly not. Every other activity on which we depend – agriculture, building, transport, manufacturing, even leisure – has been shaped by technologies that are themselves expressions of scientific understanding. It is inconceivable that medicine could have been the exception. Imagine the absurdity of living in a city like London, surrounded by computers, motor cars and every imaginable product of high technology, then developing a pain in the abdomen and visiting a doctor whose only response was to prescribe a remedy chosen because Galen, on the basis of little understanding and even less evidence, had recommended it during the middle of the second century AD.

Medicine followed the path of science because, in the search for practical benefits, it could follow no other. However medicine may change and develop in the future, it cannot abandon science. If orthodox medicine *has* made a mistake, it stems not from having embraced science, but from having sometimes embraced it to the exclusion of all else.

6 A Series of Rebellions
The development of alternative medicine

Long before the age of recorded history, there must have been shamans or medicine men who bound wounds, cooled fevers, and otherwise ministered to the medical needs of our distant ancestors. It's equally certain that they relied on a mix of magic and herbs. But to claim them exclusively as the forerunners of either today's orthodox physicians, or today's complementary practitioners would be meaningless. They represent – and their practices almost certainly encompassed – two strands of thinking, both of which exist to this day. To the extent that they used magic they were adopting a vitalist approach: a belief that living things are more than the sum of the physical and chemical forces active within them. But besides casting spells and muttering incantations, they would surely also have used physical methods of treating the body with the plant and animal remedies that all communities, however primitive, invariably accumulate. In this sense they also employed mechanistic principles of healing. They may not consciously have made any such distinction; and if they did they certainly wouldn't have conceptualized it in this way. But for many centuries these two approaches, present in medicine from the beginning, co-existed in relative harmony.

With the advent of science there came not only a theoretical basis for distinguishing between mechanist and vitalist thinking, but also a philosophical and practical need to do so. Of its nature, scientific medicine has adopted an almost entirely mechanistic approach, while its many and various alternatives are normally happy to use an alloy of the two.

As pointed out in the previous chapter, definitions of 'orthodox' and 'unorthodox' were once largely a matter of whose views carried the most clout. Science made it possible to draw distinctions on other grounds. Power and influence remained – and are still – factors in defining what is orthodox; but they are no longer the sole determinants.

That the vitalist and mechanist principles co-existed peacefully for so long is hardly surprising; in a pre-scientific era there was little basis for distinguishing between them. One of the earliest hints of the way things were to go can be found in the thirteenth century when physicians began establishing themselves in what amounted to craft guilds. Many people, of course, couldn't afford their ministrations – though given that these consisted largely of purgings, enemas, blood-lettings and the like, they may not have been missing anything of great value. The poor had to rely on whatever quacks or village 'wise women' they could find – the latter running a continual risk of being arrested by the authorities and burnt at the stake. In part this was because the vitalist strain of thinking in what they did laid them open to charges of witchcraft. This state of affairs continued through into the seventeenth century.

The rationalist mood of the Renaissance, and the emergence of science, presented some healers – herbalists, for example – with a dilemma. A part of what they did squared quite happily with the new thinking of the times; but much else was still closely tied to superstition, astrology and magic. The herbalists were not alone in finding themselves pulled in different directions.

Then, as now, the physicians themselves contributed some of the dissenting voices. Georg Ernst Stahl was a professor of medicine whose career spanned the end of the seventeenth and the beginning of the eighteenth centuries. Although trained as an orthodox physician, he rejected the learning of his day on physics, chemistry and even biology; he adopted vitalist ideas about medicine, and began to explain health and disease in terms of forces not recognized by science. But he was an exception to the steady progress being made by the mechanistic view of disease. Even practitioners of folk medicine were becoming as concerned with the content of the potions they administered as with the vitalist practices formerly associated with them. But vitalism was to re-emerge at other times, and in other forms.

Medical indignation

As each unorthodox technique appeared, the doctors responded with indignation. Their professed reasons for doing so were always the same: that patients needed protection against quacks and charlatans who would steal their money, and do them harm. Attacks based on poor results were less frequent because orthodox medicine itself had little enough to show in this respect. In hindsight it appears that even when orthodox medicine was justified in warning the public against this or that practice, it was motivated as much by professional self-interest as by public spirit.

As we've already seen, the history of orthodox medicine was anything but a linear progression. Its thinking nowadays is dominated by attempts to define the objective reality of disease; but the route towards this position was punctuated by halts, diversions and reversals. It is none the less possible, taking the long view, to describe the history of orthodox medicine in terms of a journey that started from a position of false and incomplete understanding and, over time, reached a truer and more complete one. The same can't be said of its alternatives. History, in this case, is an unconnected series of rebellions against the establishment. Some of these were motivated by radically different but honestly held ideas about the nature of health and disease; others were driven by a self-serving attempt to exploit the credulity of patients; and a few turned upon some genuine discovery that, for reasons of economics or expediency or intellectual error, was unacceptable to the establishment.

Historian Roy Porter has made a study of unorthodox medicine from the middle of the seventeenth through to the nineteenth centuries. This seems to have been a golden age for quackery. In his book *Health for Sale* he defines quacks as 'those who drummed up custom largely through self-orchestrated publicity ... whose dealings with their clients were largely one-off, and who depended heavily on vending secret nostrums.' Enterprising individuals devised countless pills, potions and other remedies for literally every illness suffered by humans, from the most trivial to the most serious. One factor in this proliferation was no doubt the emergence of new understandings in biology and medicine; these offered great scope to an imaginative entrepreneur bent on devising new treatments that sounded as if they might owe something to recent discoveries. (It should be noted that the term 'quack', as Porter uses it, doesn't have quite the pejorative connotations that usually attend that word.)

This, though, in Porter's view, was not the driving force behind quackery. What really counted was that England in this period was a place of unbridled commercialism. The free-market was all-important, and the public – consumers, as we would now describe them – was keen to test all the wares on offer, including rival treatments for disease. The medical establishment was powerless to suppress this activity, and the State made no effort to impose controls, preferring instead to tax it. Some commentators have argued that the quacks of this period are the direct ancestors of today's alternative practitioners. Interestingly, Porter disputes this view – not because the alternative practitioners of today might take offence at being seen as the descendants of mountebanks, but because he believes this to be a misreading. He points out that qualified doctors were not above resorting to their own brands of naked commercialism when it suited their purposes. Both the establishment and the quacks were engaged in much the same enterprise: drumming up whatever business they could find by whatever means they could muster. The quacks undoubtedly showed more flair for exploiting their customers' perceptions of illness. They didn't, however, do the one thing that would have entitled them to be looked on as the forerunners of today's complementary practitioners: that is, to set out genuinely different understandings of health and disease.

A different perspective

The most celebrated of those who campaigned against the quacks was the surgeon Thomas Wakeley, editor of the *Lancet*. He even founded an Anti-Quackery Society. To demonstrate that he was on the side of the angels – and not just that of the doctors – he denounced incompetence within the ranks of the medical profession itself.

If an ancestor of today's alternatives *is* to be found in this era, Roy Porter identifies it in the activities of one man: James Morison. Singled out by Thomas Wakeley for special loathing, Morison was a businessman whose own ill health had led him to seek the help of regular doctors, but without success. This experience prompted him not only to criticize the doctors, but also eventually to establish an alternative theory of illness.

He claimed that while the medical profession used many fine words and phrases, they actually knew nothing about disease. In reality, he claimed, all illness was attributable to bad blood. He summarized his beliefs in ten slogans, among which were:

The vital principle is contained in the blood;
Everything in the body is derived from the blood;
All diseases arise from the impurity of the blood;
Purgation by vegetables is the only effectual mode of eradicating disease;
From the intimate connection subsisting between the mind and the body, the health of the one must conduce to the serenity of the other.

To help people apply these theories Morison manufactured his own purgative called Vegetable Universal pills. They sold well, and Morison became wealthy.

Porter argues that while peddling a useless nostrum may

have made Morison a quack, his apparently sincere attempts to change peoples' views of health and disease made him more than this. Unlike the rest of his kind, he was advocating a real alternative to contemporary thinking about physiology and medicine. He founded an organization to champion his views, the British College of Health, and publicized them in a magazine called the *Hygeian Journal*.

Following the time of Wakeley and Morison, the quacks began to disappear. But many of the new medical theories and techniques that emerged at or shortly before this period were certainly more than mere attempts to exploit public credulity and turn a swift penny. Right or wrong they grew from the genuine beliefs of their founders that medical science had taken the wrong pathway. And as medicine rooted itself evermore firmly in the fertile soil of science, so it became possible to distinguish more meaningfully between orthodox and unorthodox medicine. From the mid-nineteenth century onwards many of these new forms of medicine began to prosper. By early Victorian times the orthodox/fringe split we recognize today was already apparent.

Mesmerism was one of the late eighteenth century inventions that triggered much medical disapproval. Franz Mesmer pioneered the development of what became known as 'animal magnetism'. This was a force said to pervade the universe, capable of acting upon living creatures, and able to be directed into an individual by a person suitably trained. Mesmer's public demonstrations were certainly spectacular, with people falling into trances as he made passes with his fingers in front of them. What Mesmer had stumbled upon was hypnosis – and the doctors of Vienna where he worked felt sufficiently threatened by his popularity to make it impossible for him to work there. Mesmer moved to Paris where once again he aroused much opposition. A commission that examined his work found it to have no value, and although the phrase 'animal magnetism' is familiar enough, mesmerism as such failed to prosper. But its successor, hypnotism, remains alive and well.

Homeopathy and osteopathy

Homeopathy also made the doctors angry – an effect it can still have a century and a half later. It was devised by Dr Samuel Hahnemann towards the end of the eighteenth century. His basic idea – that 'like cures like' – was inspired when he noticed that Peruvian bark, a standard cure for malaria (and a source of quinine, which was why it worked) itself produced feverish symptoms when taken by someone who is healthy. Because he was anxious about the safety of the materials he was testing – often on himself – he would use them in dilute form. In so doing he discovered the other main characteristic of homeopathy: that diluting its various active ingredients tended not to diminish the body's response to them, but to increase it. After years of observation and testing he published his findings in a book called *Homeopathic materia medica*. Although modern homeopaths do not labour the point, Hahnemann himself held explicitly vitalist views of homeopathy. He wrote of the body in health as being ruled by a vital force that generates harmony; in sickness, on the other hand, the vital force becomes deranged, the result being the unpleasant sensations of which we then become aware.

This was all too much for the doctors of Hahnemann's native Austria. They took him to court and even tried to have homeopathy banned. Orthodox medicine mounted a number of other assaults during the next century. When the General Medical Council was set up in Britain in 1858, doctors had great hopes of being able to use it to outlaw homeopathy; indeed, as originally conceived, the Council would have been able to strike off any doctor for using it. But this element of its constitution was abandoned. In the long run, of course, homeopathy survived and is now the most secure and in many countries the most 'respectable' branch of complementary medicine. In Britain, for example, it is practised by doctors with orthodox qualifications, and even enshrined – albeit on a token scale – within the NHS.

Another source of irritation to conventional medicine were

the spinal manipulators: the osteopaths and the chiropractors. Both began in the United States, in areas where doctors were in short supply and much of the healing was still in the hands of bone-setters. Andrew Still, who founded osteopathy, was a farmer, a healer and (significantly) a mechanic who believed that because man was made in the image of God, the design of the human body must be perfect. Disease, he reasoned, must be the result of imperfections that had crept in, and which could be overcome by adjusting the body in various ways. He devised a system of manipulation, which he announced in 1874. He tried to interest doctors, but failed. Chiropractic suffered much the same experience. Devised by a grocer called D. D. Palmer it began as a variant of osteopathy.

Both treatments might have achieved the acceptance of doctors if they had confined themselves to disorders of the spine and its associated joints and muscles. But both, on the basis of elaborate and largely fallacious theory, made claims to be universal therapies. America's and, later, other countries' medical bodies mounted the usual attempts at suppression, but again failed. Osteopathy and chiropractic eventually gained a degree of acceptance by quietly ditching much of their founders' original theory, and by making less extravagant claims about the range of disorders in which their therapies might be beneficial.

Vitalism again

A strong reaffirmation of the vitalist thread emerged at the beginning of this century when an American, Dr Albert Abrams, invented radionics. With its uncompromising reliance on extrasensory perception and other forces more familiar to psychics than to physicians, this treatment too got under the skin of the doctors. In Britain it led to the 'black box' investigation – the black box being the name commonly used to describe the instruments used by radionics practitioners. A committee of doctors chaired by Lord (as he later became) Horder set up a test in which the operator of the black box had to use his equipment to identify tissues, chemicals and various other objects that he wasn't allowed to see. In this, and in a subsequent test, the equipment confounded the doctors by performing exactly as its inventor claimed it would! Thus wrong-footed, the medical establishment had no option but to back off. Despite this triumph, radionics has never penetrated far beyond the fringe of the fringe.

The rapid progress and manifest success of orthodox medicine during the first half of the twentieth century continued to present unorthodox practitioners with a problem: why should the public take notice of them and their wares when so enchanted with the fruits of science? In Britain, the post-war emergence of the National Health Service created a further obstacle: orthodox treatment would henceforth be free at the time of need; alternative treatments would have to be paid for. Some groups, such as the herbalists, might have been allowed into the NHS – but only at the price of working under the control of doctors. They preferred to remain out in the cold, but independent.

Around the beginning of the 1960s, the fortunes of the unorthodox practitioners began to change. The then editor of the *Spectator*, Brian Inglis, commissioned a review of what was happening in unorthodox medicine. Inspired by the fringe events that were growing up around the official Edinburgh Festival, Inglis and Geoffrey Murray (the author of the piece) devised the term 'fringe medicine'. This eventually gave way to the more dignified 'alternative medicine'. One of the first therapies to profit by this rediscovery was acupuncture – in part, no doubt, because its oriental origins made an interest in it highly fashionable. The thalidomide tragedy gave a boost to herbalism, its practitioners claiming that their preparations, unlike those of the drug industry, were free of side effects. By now the floodgates were open, and complementary therapies, as they came to be known ('alternative' gave an impression of competition with orthodox medicine), began to proliferate.

Boom time for alternatives

How many complementary therapies are now available is difficult to estimate because some overlap each other, and new variants keep on appearing. One of the free local newspapers that drops weekly through my own home letterbox, a modest enough affair called the *Camden New Journal*, regularly includes a page and a half on health matters, some two-thirds of it comprising advertisements for local practitioners. One issue, chosen at random, offered the following choice: osteopathy; cranial osteopathy; acupuncture; aromatherapy; Alexander technique; homeopathy; massage; shiatsu; iridology; chiropractic; herbalism; meditation; healing; transformational workshops; holistic reflexology; kinesiology; bodywork; colonics; hypnosis; 'skills for the new age'; and 'divine love'. Given the anarchic state of complementary medicine it is difficult to estimate the cost of all this activity. One 1985 figure put it at upwards of £150 million in fees to practitioners, with perhaps another £100 million being spent on associated medicines and the like. The number of therapists has been growing at the rate of 10 per cent annually, and as public interest shows no signs of abating, this growth is likely to be maintained.

Why this proliferation? Some of the reasons are positive. Many people, for example, are attracted to complementary therapies because they're perceived as 'natural'. The rise of the green movement reflects a desire to live in harmony with nature instead of living continually at odds with it. In a world crowded with aircraft, motor cars, cities and television sets such a yearning is as understandable as it is, sadly, unattainable – or at least attainable only to a limited degree. In these circumstances, the concept of what *is* 'natural' has taken some rather odd forms. In truth, it has been inflated in such a way that more people can enjoy the consolation of doing or having something that they can comfortably think of as 'natural', even if the term has been rendered virtually meaningless. As far as medicine is concerned, it is not immediately obvious why curing a headache by sticking needles into the skin should be thought of as more 'natural' than swallowing an aspirin. But then complementary medicine is less about what you do than the way in which you do it. And there is no disputing that most unorthodox practitioners *do* operate quite differently from most doctors.

The flight from science

Green ideas are not to be disparaged; in so far as they are about finding ways of living that are indefinitely sustainable, they represent all our hopes for the future. But the rise of complementary medicine has not been fuelled solely or even mainly by such positive thoughts. Much of it has stemmed from a disillusionment with orthodox medicine – itself part of a larger and wider disillusionment with science, and the products of science. First, then, the broader context: this 'flight from science'.

Although we live in a world that has been shaped by science and technology, a great many of us remain remarkably ill-informed about it, and the discoveries it has led to. A poll carried out among British people in 1990 revealed that one-third of us think that the Sun goes round the Earth, more than half believe that antibiotics kill viruses as well as bacteria, and one in seven are under the impression that milk contaminated with radioactivity can be rendered safe by boiling it. In truth our attitudes towards science are paradoxical; although the same survey showed that four out of five people claim to be interested in scientific, medical and technological advances, there is a widespread suspicion of science and, among a small but not negligible minority, a deep hostility to it.

The most obvious reason for this antagonism is to be found in the technological horrors that our century has bred: atomic, chemical and biological weapons and other military applications of science; chemical and radioactive pollution; and the many other varieties of environmental destruction to which technology has contributed. Science has brought us nuclear energy, a source of power generation that was once worshipped, and is now disliked and feared beyond all reason. Then there are agricultural chemicals, food additives, genetic engineering... but there seems little point in adding to the list. Enough to say that science is judged responsible in some measure for the adverse consequences of all these things. Peoples' attitudes towards it are shaped accordingly.

Science is also thought to be cruel – witness vivisection. Philosophically it is held to be dehumanizing, to remove the mystery from everyday experience. Scientists are not infrequently derided as soulless. There are, of course, whole areas of human experience to which science has no direct relevance. It is not necessary to understand *why* York Minster or a Beethoven symphony evoke such deep feelings. And of the few academic scientists who might take a professional interest in trying to account for our response to music or architecture, fewer still would sit through the choral movement of Beethoven's Ninth wondering how the nerve cells of their brains are transforming the 'Ode to Joy' into emotional responses. Like the rest of us they are content to embrace the emotion without wondering at that particular moment why they feel what they're feeling.

Although there is, as I say, no practical necessity to explain such things, someone may eventually be able to construct an explanation framed in terms of neurophysiology and psychology. Would this devalue such experiences? Not at all. The claim that acquiring a better understanding of something devalues it is at odds with experience. In truth, to know a thing better is usually to value it more. To understand the theory of evolution is not to cease wondering at the beauty of living things; to understand a fraction of what's happening inside a single cell is to find a new respect for the integrated workings of the whole body. And yet the view persists that science is narrow and blinkered and antithetical to human values.

The world is, without doubt, full of unpleasant things, some of them the products of a technology informed by and rooted in science. The fault, though, lies not in the science or the technology, but much closer to home: in those who command and deploy it. In ourselves.

Suspicion of orthodox medicine

Against this background of a rumbling suspicion of science and all its works, the image of medicine too has become corroded in the past couple of decades. The fact that it owes so much to science automatically damns it in the eyes of some critics. And the increasing domination of medicine by technology has disturbed many patients – often justifiably. The gratuitous use of life support systems to keep the Spanish dictator Franco alive was a classic example of the perversion of medicine made possible by technology. The further accusation levelled at all sorts of medical techniques, including psychosurgery, transplantation, and in vitro fertilization is that all treat human beings as if they were machines. Some treatments, however well-intentioned, are of their nature distressing. Anti-cancer drugs, for example, may have effects as unpleasant as the tumour they're intended to attack.

Medicine does, of course, have its acknowledged disasters. The side effects of Thalidomide were horrific. That episode, and several since, have bred a not uncommon suspicion of all drug therapy. There is, undeniably, a price to be paid for modern medicine. A study carried out at one university hospital in the United States found that more than a third of 815 patients admitted consecutively to a general medical ward had an iatrogenic illness: that is, a condition caused by something given or done to them by a doctor. In almost 10 per cent of cases the incident threatened life or produced disability. In 2 per cent of the 815 patients, iatrogenic illness probably contributed to their deaths.

And then there's the cost of medicine. In America it's over 10 per cent of GNP and still rising – out of control, say some critics. Opponents of modern medicine such as Ivan Illich have seized on these things and used them to mount a frontal assault. Nor have the doctors helped themselves by consciously or otherwise raising peoples' expectations of a cure for all forms of disease. Twenty years on, when the promised treatments have failed to materialize, people may forget what *has* been achieved and think only of what hasn't. Yet another stick with which to beat the doctors. And all the while there is the siren voice of complementary medicine hinting or whispering or even shouting that it can offer every bit as much benefit, but without the penalties. It can't, of course. Like orthodox medicine it has its limitations. And advocates of scientific medicine would argue that if complementary therapies have fewer side effects, it is because they also have fewer beneficial ones as well. The debate will continue. But to reject the notion of scientific medicine as a panacea, and then to put complementary medicine on the same pedestal would be to repeat the error.

There is, then, no single reason why complementary medicine has become so popular. But a disenchantment with science in general, and orthodox scientific medicine in particular – however unfair or ill-judged at least some of the accusations may be – is surely at the heart of it.

Recent developments

In recent years, the increasing confidence of some of the leading complementary practitioners has encouraged them to test their remedies sufficiently rigorously to merit publication of the results in orthodox medical journals such as the *Lancet*. Homeopaths have critically evaluated their techniques in a range of conditions, including arthritis, fibrositis and hay fever. A review of the literature carried out in 1991 identified more than 100 published controlled trials of homeopathy, and found that while its case could not be taken as proved, the balance of the evidence lay in favour of accepting that it works. Acupuncture is another therapy that has embarked with some success on the path towards scientific respectability.

A trial of chiropractic organized by the Medical Research Council illustrated how rewarding it can be to carry out scientifically acceptable studies. The patients who took part in this research project all suffered from low back pain of a type that is both common and difficult to manage. Each underwent a preliminary assessment to check that their conditions were of the sort which chiropractors might deem suitable for this type of treatment. Half the patients were then referred for chiropractic; the remainder received whatever therapy their local hospitals routinely provided for back trouble of this kind. After a predetermined period all the patients were reassessed. By and large, the group treated by the chiropractors had done rather better than those who had been dealt with by conventional hospital methods.

Both the chiropractors and the doctors seem to have been reasonably satisfied with this preliminary exercise in collaboration, and more such will surely follow. But the investigation of the unorthodox or the unexpected is not always carried off quite so harmoniously. The Benveniste affair is a case in point.

During the late 1980s Jacques Benveniste, a biologist employed by the French equivalent of the Medical Research Council, was working with a type of white blood cells called basophils. These contain a large number of coarse granules containing various chemicals, including histamine. Under certain circumstances basophils 'degranulate': that is, they release the contents of their granules. The 'basophil degranulation test' is one of the standard methods of investigating patients thought to be suffering from hay fever and other such hypersensitivity reactions. The details of this test are irrelevant; the point is that basophil degranulation is a well-studied reaction, used routinely in laboratories around the world.

As with most biological responses, degranulation is not an all-or-none phenomenon; the more of the material there is in the test system that is serving to trigger the degranulation response, the more degranulation will occur. Benveniste was working with very small concentrations of his triggering agents – so small that there should have been insufficient material present to have any effect. But Benveniste claimed that he *was* getting a reaction – provided the test tubes holding the triggering agents were vibrated vigorously between each dilution. To anyone familiar with homeopathy, this will sound familiar. An essential part of the methodology of preparing homeopathic remedies is to shake them vigorously – succussion, to use the technical term – between each dilution. Without this shaking, so it's claimed, the remedies are not effective.

Homeopaths were delighted when a research report describing the work and its findings was published in 1988 in the journal *Nature*, the Bible of orthodoxy as far as scientific publishing is concerned. However, *Nature*'s editor also printed what amounted to a disclaimer: an odd thing to have done. Journals like *Nature* publish only reports that have been refereed by independent experts. If they approve the work, all well and good; if they don't, the report is rejected and that is the end of the matter. Odder still was the editor's decision to investigate the working methods used in Benveniste's laboratory – a visit that was made *after* publication of his report. The visiting team comprised a scientist familiar with the detection of scientific fraud, a magician with an interest in exposing how allegedly paranormal phenomena can be duplicated by sleight of hand, and the editor himself. Having inspected Benveniste's laboratory, his colleagues and their methods, the team pronounced itself dissatisfied. The work that had already been published in *Nature* was in effect rejected retrospectively.

This whole unsatisfactory affair served to reinforce everyone's prejudices. To many orthodox scientists it was further evidence that homeopathy is nonsense, and anyone trying to account for it in terms of conventional scientific thinking must be a knave or a fool. To many practitioners of complementary medicine the saga confirmed that orthodox science is so deeply prejudiced that attempts at co-operation are pointless. A sad conclusion.

Bristol Cancer Help Centre

Even sadder was the affair of the Bristol Cancer Help Centre (BCHC). Set up in 1979 to offer various forms of alternative therapy to patients with cancer, its failure to assess its own effectiveness attracted criticism from doctors – many of whom were anyway sceptical about its treatment regime. This included a diet of raw vegetables designed to 'detoxify' the body, and so boost the chances of cancer regression; attempts to stimulate the immune system into mounting a more effective attack against the tumour; and efforts to create a harmonious balance between each patient's mind, body and spirit. In 1986 the centre felt it should meet the challenge of its critics. It asked a group of eminent doctors and scientists to advise on how best to evaluate its results. Two studies were planned: one was to investigate survival following treatment at the centre; the other was to find out whether it improved patients' quality of life, irrespective of whether it affected their survival.

At the time of writing, only the survival study has been published. It compared patients with breast cancer who had and had not been treated at Bristol. The results, when they appeared, were shattering for staff at the centre. Although the members of the independent research team who carried out the work had expected to find no difference between the two groups, they actually found survival to be poorer among the group who had undergone the Bristol treatment. The researchers themselves were at a loss to explain their findings. But they added that in the light of evidence that the outlook of women with breast cancer can influence their prognosis, it was conceivable that something about the psychology of the sort of patients attracted to the Bristol Centre might account for their relatively poor survival.

In subsequent weeks it emerged that the two groups of patients who had been compared were not strictly identical. One of the reasons for this was that the practice of randomly allocating patients to treatment or no treatment – a standard element of such comparisons – had not been acceptable to staff at the centre. When one of the Bristol doctors wrote to the *Lancet* listing this among the criticisms of the trial, he provoked a response from two orthodox specialists.

> It does seem rather brazen of the BCHC to claim that the study was 'seriously flawed' because it was non-randomized, since the initial recommendation to them was that a randomized study was much the best way forward. On a lighter note, it reminded us both of the apocryphal story of the Jewish boy who slew both his parents, then threw himself at the mercy of the court on the grounds that he was now an orphan. Such *chutzpah*!

Neither of the authors of that letter, Professors Michael Baum and Jeffrey Tobias, would describe themselves as great friends of complementary therapy – which may account for the hint of triumphalism in their letter. But putting this to one side, they go on to testify from personal experience that the atmosphere at the Bristol Centre induces a feeling of well-being.

> The important question is whether this translates into a genuine long-term improvement in the quality of life. This possibility clearly needs to be subjected to critical review since it is equally possible to construct an alternative hypothesis – namely that a short-lived sense of well-being and control may deteriorate when the BCHC regime starts to become a daily reminder that the person remains a cancer patient, and not like other people. Daily ritual and eccentric diets have been in use for millennia to separate out one class of human beings from their fellows. This may be fine for religion, but is it right for cancer?

There is no doubt that making a disease the centre of your life has the effect of concentrating the mind; but they are right to query whether an emphasis of this kind is necessarily beneficial. This is especially so when a therapy emphasizes that an individual has the power to help him or herself. The unspoken codicil to this proposition is that individuals have only themselves to blame for falling ill in the first place. Besides suffering the misery of the disease itself, some people are left with the added despondency of feeling that it is all their own fault. Some orthodox clinicians dealing with cancer patients are angry about the side effects of this attribution of personal responsibility. They claim to have come across patients who are deeply distressed as a result of treatments based on this premise.

One of the more recent and most rarified preoccupations of those interested in complementary medicine is an attempt to demonstrate that some of its apparently unscientific claims and theories are actually in line with modern physics. Quantum theory in particular is often invoked for these purposes. To start dissecting such claims lies beyond the scope of this book. It should, though, be noted that the laws of ordinary, Newtonian physics only break down when dealing with objects that are galactically huge, sub-atomically small, or travelling at very high speed. For day to day purposes – in this instance when dealing with cells, tissues, organs and whole human beings – the ordinary laws of Newtonian physics continue to work perfectly satisfactorily.

It is often assumed that if complementary therapy is effective, it ought to be integrated within the National Health Service, and become another component of the regular treatment package. There is, though, a potential drawback to such a step. Suppose that much – or at any rate part – of the benefit of some complementary medicine stems from the very fact that its techniques *are* unorthodox: that they are outside the system and therefore in some way 'special'. Recall a phenomenon mentioned elsewhere in this book: the Hawthorne effect, the tendency of people to perform well simply because attention is being paid to them. The feeling that a treatment is in some way 'special' could exercise a powerful placebo effect – which might be lost if this or that complementary procedure became just another treatment. This is an objection that will have to be taken on board when the time comes to consider how far it is feasible to integrate orthodox and unorthodox medicine.

PART THREE: One Medicine

7 Who Are the Healers Now?

The key differences between orthodox and alternative medicine

As the cases and consultations described in Chapter 4 revealed, there is a marked difference in the way that doctors and complementary practitioners relate to their patients. It arises from the equally marked differences in the ways they view themselves. Most herbalists, reflexologists and naturopaths would describe their role, in some sense or other, as that of a healer. This is not a term that most doctors nowadays would use; indeed, many would feel a certain degree of embarrassment at being so described. And even doctors who countenance the idea might feel the use of the term 'healer' to be slightly pompous.

At first sight this is odd because doctors are the lineal descendants of generations of individuals who would happily have accepted the label 'healer'. To understand why doctors have come to feel uncomfortable with the word, you have to recall the changes that have overtaken medicine during the past hundred years.

Throughout most of the history of doctoring, the key element – albeit unrealized – in the attempt to help patients has been the doctors themselves. Until quite recently, knowledge of the human body and how it worked was rudimentary. Some of the later physicians may have possessed a modest number of instruments, and a selection of medications; but the whole lot could have been bundled into a few cupboards, and the practice of medicine required no special setting or buildings.

Think now of the present decade: of the sorts of things that doctors can do, and the facilities they require to do them. Think of the intensive care unit, the epitome of the technological medicine of this century.

The intensive care unit is an unnerving place. The patients often seem – and often are – closer to death than to life. They are surrounded by flashing, bleeping machinery with dials and paper traces that register and record their heart rate, their breathing, and other vital functions. They are linked to the machinery by tubes and catheters that variously feed them, maintain their fluid balance, pump air into their lungs and remove their waste products. The lighting is usually bright and frequently harsh and there is a constant background noise from the instrumentation and its associated power and cooling supplies. There are nurses around, but they are busy and often stressed, and their first concern is not so much the patients as the equipment on which those patients' lives depend. It is a dehumanizing environment in which the role of the medical and nursing staff is primarily that of highly-skilled technicians.

Ubiquitous technology

The intensive care unit may be the most extreme example of technological medicine, but it is not the only part of the hospital in which instruments and machinery are the most prominent feature. The X-ray equipment in diagnostic radiology departments grows evermore elaborate; so does the apparatus for treating cancer using radiotherapy. Change and development are everywhere. There are whole new hospital departments reliant on techniques that a few decades ago didn't even exist. Lasers can be deployed to weld a detached retina, burn through a blocked coronary artery, or blast the pigment out of an unwanted tattoo. Elsewhere in the hospital there are instruments producing beams of ultrasound that allow the doctor to measure the speed of the blood flowing through a vessel, or discern the unborn foetus moving in the womb. Machines that generate powerful shock waves can be used to smash kidney stones into tiny fragments that will then pass out of the body in the urine.

Surgery, too, has been undergoing a radical change. The traditional and bloody but simple approach – in which the surgeon slices his way through skin and muscle to reach the internal organs – is giving way to surgery through the endoscope. This is a telescope designed for peering inside the body. Slid through the mouth and down the oesophagus it allows the doctor to view the stomach and even the first section of the small intestine stretching beyond it. A similar instrument inserted through the anus reveals the interior of the rectum, and the lining of the large bowel. A slimmer version of the endoscope, introduced into the urethra, makes it possible to visualize the interior of the bladder. And by making a small puncture wound in the skin of the abdomen, the surgeon can create a new and easily repaired orifice through which to scrutinize other organs within the body cavity.

Being able to see these things has, by itself, proved a valuable aid to diagnosis; and there's increasing enthusiasm for operating by this route. Specially designed instruments can be slipped through tubes just a few millimetres in diameter. Using the endoscope, the doctor can both see the target organ, and manipulate it. Enlarged prostates can be trimmed to normal size; small tumours on the bowel lining can be lassooed using a kind of wire hook and snipped off; and stomach ulcers can be sealed using laser beams fired through the endoscope. Procedures that can't be done under direct vision can often be controlled by using an X-ray viewing system. The fine instruments show up as shadows on the screen, and the surgeon performs his work as though manipulating Javanese shadow puppets. More and more operations are being done using these 'minimally invasive' methods, as they are known.

As startling in its way as the evolution of surgery has been the development of drug therapy. A glimpse of the storeroom in any local pharmacy is enough to reveal how many medicines the doctor has to choose from – and what's on show is only a fraction of what's available. To get some idea of the extent of our ingenuity and enthusiasm for chemically influencing our bodies, flip through any standard pharmacopoeia. The range is startling. The process of drug development too has changed. The time-honoured approach was trial and error; indeed, testing large numbers of compounds in the hope of stumbling on physiological effects with therapeutic potential is still a fertile source of new agents. But as more is understood about the nature of disease at cellular and molecular levels, chemists engaged on drug development are gradually learning to proceed by design.

If the biologist knows, for example, that such and such a physiological process is controlled by this or that hormone, he may identify the receptor to which that hormone attaches, and through which it switches on the process. Using the familiar analogy of a lock and a key – in which the receptor is the lock, and the hormone the key – the chemist can then synthesize a new molecule that is structurally similar to the hormone, but not identical. With luck, this molecule will fit neatly into the receptor, but *not* turn it on. It is as if you'd sealed up the keyhole of the front door, so preventing anyone else inserting another key and opening it.

The most familiar example of this ploy is in the action of the beta-blockers, a type of drug used for treating, amongst other things, angina. The speed at which the heart beats is under the control of nerves with endings bearing what are designated beta-receptors. These respond specifically to a hormone, adrenalin, which is released by the adrenal glands. Beta-blocking drugs do just what their name implies: they attach themselves to the beta-receptors and block them, but *without* activating them. The keyhole is sealed off. With its nerve endings now isolated from the stimulating effect of any adrenalin present in the blood, the heart slows; it beats less hard, does less work, demands less

WHO ARE THE HEALERS NOW?

oxygen – and so no longer causes pain. The angina has been controlled.

Increasing numbers of these 'designer drugs' are now finding their way out of the laboratory and into the pharmacy. The hope is that with increased understanding of the chemical and hormonal control mechanisms operating inside the body, the trend will continue and even accelerate.

This handful of examples of what has been achieved by applying science to medicine could be multiplied a hundred times over, but the point is made. Scientists have become extremely good at understanding how the body works, and putting that understanding to therapeutic use. Medical technologists and engineers are forever designing new instruments and equipment that make it possible to do things, from open-heart surgery to hip replacement, that were once unimaginable. And underlying all this – indeed, the inspiration for much of it – is a machine model of the human body and how it works.

The doctor as body technician

Given this state of affairs, is it surprising that medical staff have a tendency to behave as if they're car mechanics – or body technicians? Admittedly it is only the hospital specialists who spend a significant part of their working day surrounded by the instrumentation; who spend, as it were, their time in the repair shop where the hardware is taken apart and reassembled. But the GP is as conscious as the brain surgeon of the things that can now be done to or for the body, and is affected by that knowledge. Indeed, it would be surprising if day-by-day doctoring failed to reflect these extraordinary developments. There would be little point in the gadgets and the gizmos if no one knew they existed, and no patients were referred for treatment with them.

The notion of medicine as body technology has become an in-built part of the training of doctors. Fanciful thoughts that students may have of training to become healers are soon knocked out of them as they wrestle with the latest findings of neurochemistry and immunology. But although most patients recognize that doctors have a technical function to fulfil, and applaud them for what they do, patients need and want more than this.

Doctors are not, of course, the only people offering a service from whom we expect something beyond mere efficiency; but in fairness to the medical profession, we ask considerably more of them than we do of most other trades and professions. They see us when we are most confused, most distressed, most anxious, and sometimes in need of much, much more than small acts of politeness and friendliness. For years doctors have been complaining that they have had to take on tasks that once fell to others. The decline of religion, they say, has left them having to fulfil the priestly duties of offering comfort to the bereaved, guidance to the spiritually confused, and a confessional ear to anyone with a burdened conscience. The contraction from extended to nuclear families has meant that fewer relatives are on hand to undertake these duties.

Moreover, there is a distinct mismatch between the training given to doctors – mainly concerned with the treatment of physical disease – and the reality of what they will encounter when they start work, especially if they go into general practice. A detailed knowledge of the biochemistry of blood clotting doesn't help a great deal when trying to support a teenager coping with an unwanted pregnancy, or to comfort an agoraphobic old lady whose canary has just died. It is true that medical students do now receive some preparation for the shock of dealing with patients who are also people, but the greater part of their training is still in applied human biology.

Oliver Sacks, the neurologist best known for his book *Awakenings*, has pointed to this loss of humanity in medicine. *Awakenings* is his account of the effects of the drug L-dopa on patients suffering from the Parkinsonian symptoms brought on by Encephalitis Lethargica, otherwise known as the sleepy sickness. He comments on the vast scientific literature about this topic:

One mulls over whole libraries of papers, couched in the 'objective', styleless style *de rigeur* in neurology; one's head buzzes with facts, figures, lists, schedules, inventories, calculations, ratings, quotients, indices, statistics, formulae, graphs, and whatnot; everything 'calculated, cast up, balanced, and proved' in a manner which would have delighted the heart of a Thomas Gradgrind. And nowhere, *nowhere*, does one find any colour, reality, or warmth; nowhere any residue of the living experience; nowhere any impression or picture of what it *feels* like to have Parkinsonism, to receive L-dopa and to be totally transformed. If ever there was a subject which needed a non-mechanical treatment, it is this one; but one looks in vain for life in these papers; they are the ugliest exemplars of production-line medicine: everything living, everything human, pounded, pulverized, atomized, quantized, and otherwise 'processed' out of existence.

On a more mundane level I well remember one particular visit to a GP I was registered with. I was the last patient at the end of the busy day; knowing that I have an interest in doctoring, he thought me a suitable recipient for his end-of-a-bad-day thoughts. 'Every patient I've had this evening just wants to talk,' he groaned. 'They all want to go on about their free-floating anxiety.'

On one level I could sympathize. Many doctors get their biggest kicks from diagnosis. Here is a patient with a certain set of signs and symptoms, let me see if I can crack this puzzle, and identify the illness. If the diagnosis proves successful, there may even be a pay-off in terms of prescribing a cure to which the patient responds by getting well. Given this ideal, how frustrating to be confronted with a succession of obviously unhappy people who have only vague signs of organic illness – or even none at all – who can't say very precisely what they think is the matter, and who really want the one thing you haven't the time for: talk.

Patient dissatisfaction

The area of medicine in which patient dissatisfaction first manifested itself in an organized way was childbirth. To many women the very idea that a healthy woman giving birth should be treated as if she were a sick patient needing medical help was precisely what was wrong with childbirth in hospital. Some key phrases began to crop up: 'choice in childbirth', for example. If a woman wanted her partner with her during labour, why shouldn't she? If she wanted to give birth squatting, or in a darkened room, what right had the obstetrician and the midwife to say she couldn't? The arguments in favour of this 'demedicalization' of birth acquired a powerful momentum. Sometimes, of course, they became absurd. A few campaigners appeared to believe that the process of birth was more important than the outcome – the newborn infant.

The doctors responded to all this by quoting statistics about risk, and figures on perinatal death rates. The women argued that this response was just a smokescreen put up to prevent what the doctors really wanted to avoid: the loss of their power to insist that obstetrics be arranged in a way that suited them, not the women.

It would be wrong to say that medicine is now, or has been for many years, unaware of consumer dissatisfaction. Doctors do discuss these things; the more enlightened members of the profession have been to the barricades on the side of the patients, guiding them towards a clearer understanding of what it is that they themselves really want. Yet for all the GP training initiatives, the encounter groups, the role play, and the theories about the nature of general practice, a great many patients seem to go on making the same complaint about their doctors. He's not sympathetic; he just doesn't seem to have the time.

One response is to say that people are simply asking too much of medicine. Maybe so; but to leave it at that isn't a great deal of help to the patients. The profession's current response to such complaints is, laudably, to keep GP list sizes as short as possible, and to experiment with new training initiatives intended to turn out doctors more attuned to peoples' needs.

Somehow, though, it is difficult to believe that this more-of-much-the-same approach is likely to succeed. Perhaps what is needed is an altogether more radical change. And there is another and totally different way of tackling this apparently intractable problem of patient dissatisfaction. It lies in recognizing that anyone who wants to train and function successfully as a body technician in an age when our grasp of body technology is advancing so rapidly is taking on a full time task. Medicine began sub-dividing itself into different specialities because no one person could grasp everything there is to know about every field of medicine. Could the time be coming when even the generalist in medicine should recognize that knowing enough to be an effective body technician leaves too little room for other forms of healing?

I raise this possibility with some trepidation; I have no wish to provide doctors with a justification for treating their patients with any less humanity than they do at present. My suggestion is not that they throw off all responsibility for the non-material elements of healing, but that they recognize that certain ways of achieving this end may require more time than they can afford, and the acquisition of skills that they haven't got and for which they may anyway not be suited. I'll return to this in a later chapter. In the meantime, there is much to be learned by considering the way in which complementary practitioners go about their work.

Complementary practitioners

By comparison with their counterparts in orthodox medicine, complementary practitioners rely less on technology. Chiropractors use X-rays to check the alignment of their patients' bones and joints; and medically qualified homeopaths, having a foot in both camps, accept much of what orthodox medicine can offer, and use the technology accordingly. Otherwise, though, the equipment tends to be simple – the acupuncturist's needles, the aromatherapist's essential oils – or, in the case of relaxation, massage and breath training, almost non-existent. Even the most technically sophisticated complementary therapist doesn't need anything as complicated and expensive as the hospitals that are now essential for the practice of much orthodox medicine.

The very fact that they have so limited a technological armamentarium means that complementary practitioners are free to concentrate more of their attention on the patient. And this they do with zeal. First consultations may last as long as forty minutes, much of this time spent taking a full history. While doctors will be most interested in obtaining specific details of whatever disorder has brought the patient to the surgery, the complementary therapist's questioning is likely to range far and wide. Work, home life, diet, state of mind, relationships, ways of relaxing, the ups and downs of health in the past; all this, and much else will be queried and recorded. The object of such an interrogation is to give the therapist a rounded picture of the patient: mental, physical and social. It is one of the tenets of most forms of complementary medicine that illness is an individual affair; no two sick people have exactly the same problem, and the way of dealing with whatever is the matter is to put the symptoms into their wider context.

This, of course, is the famous holistic principle. In recent years the word has been both over and incorrectly used. It has become a synonym for complementary medicine, which it is not. It is possible to use acupuncture to alleviate a particular pain without knowing anything more about the patient than a doctor might when prescribing an analgesic drug. Few complementary practitioners *would* work in this way; but there's certainly nothing to stop them doing so. It is also true that much good orthodox medicine is holistic in the sense that the doctor is interested in more than the specific pain that has brought the patient to the surgery, and wishes to know how the pain has affected that person's life, how well he or she is coping with it, and whether removing the pain will by itself get to the root of the problem. The main difference between the two forms of medicine is over the relevance of the detail. Most doctors would argue that collecting as much detail as complementary therapists are apt to do is a waste of time, and because time is in short supply in conventional medicine, they don't do it.

Most complementary practitioners spend at least four or five times as long with their patients as do most doctors. They regard this as indispensible. Patients, too, appreciate it. As they're usually paying for the service, they have a right to expect a more leisurely pace. Orthodox medicine, too, of course, is available in longer sessions – at a price. The simple fact of spending longer with a practitioner affects the kind of patient–therapist relationship that is created.

Diagnosis is another area of distinct difference. There is, naturally, an overlap; some complementary practitioners will use terms that differ little from those of the doctor. But others speak in ways that are, as far as orthodox medicine is concerned, meaningless. They will talk of 'energy flows being out of balance', of various 'inner states' that need to be 'adjusted', of subtle upsets in body function or vitality. Some even resort to paranormal phenomena and categorize patients by disturbances of an aura that is visible only to those with the sensitivity required to perceive it. Treatment is decided on the basis of whatever manoeuvre is necessary to correct these various signs.

What the patients want

Orthodox medicine looks upon such things as, at best, unproven or, at worst, gibberish. Many of the words have mystical connotations. The odd thing – particularly irritating to doctors, I'm sure – is that many people get more out of being told that their 'inner being is out of balance' than they do out of knowing that their haemoglobin level is low. The latter may mean little to them; but even sceptics will recognize the former as a kind of metaphorical description of the feelings that may have driven them to seek help in the first place.

Complementary treatments themselves are so diverse that it is sometimes difficult to be sure that a newly-announced therapy isn't a spoof. Almost anything you can imagine doing to, with, or for another person is, or has been advocated as beneficial. And while virtually all orthodox medicine is underpinned by the same theoretical foundations, complementary medicine is the product of many philosophies, or of none. A bewildering variety of sometimes contradictory ideas co-exist, their various exponents apparently untroubled by what, to the outsider, seems hopelessly chaotic.

Complementary therapies do, however, have a few features in common. A number of them – massage, chiropractic, osteopathy, reflexology, faith healing, etc. – usually involve physical contact between patient and practitioner. Aside from the occasional handshake, the only touch you're likely to get from many GPs is the light pressure of a chilly stethoscope. And that, of course, is for diagnosis, not treatment. Most of the treatments of modern medicine simply don't require the doctor to put his hands on you. This is entirely understandable but sad, because physical contact is a valuable means of healing; something we all learn during early childhood.

A feature that even more complementary therapies have in common is their emphasis on participation in treatment. Orthodox medicine generally treats the patient as a passive recipient of whatever the doctor thinks best: 'doctor's orders', as the saying has it. The doctor writes out a prescription or issues whatever other instructions he or she deems necessary, and the patients do as they are told. With few exceptions there is little attempt to discuss what might be the most appropriate course of action. Frequently, too, the remedies on offer from complementary practitioners demand more of the patient than swallowing a pill. Dietary change and specific exercises are commonly part of the treatment. The patient may be asked to change the way he or she lives. Some therapies require patients to be despatched on what amount to voyages of self-discovery in which they have to trace the roots of their own illness and find out for themselves why they became unhealthy. This is demanding stuff; very different from the 'pill for every ill' philosophy that often seems to characterize conventional medical thinking.

The limits of achievement

Most complementary medicine recognizes no set limits to what it can achieve. Orthodox medicine, confronted with a patient whose tumour has given rise to more secondaries than any anti-cancer drug can deal with, is likely to view this as the end of the road. In the past, doctors were inclined to think that having done everything they could to save a patient's life, but failed, they had discharged their responsibility. The advent of the hospice movement, and a greater concern within medicine for quality as well as quantity of life, has done much to change things.

Complementary medicine is less concerned with the struggle to save life at all costs. Its practitioners are willing to take on patients for whom the doctors have said there is no hope. The majority – though not all – of such people do indeed die. The difference is that most complementary practitioners are less likely to prejudge their chances of success; they are more inclined to press ahead whatever with an optimistic zeal. AIDS patients are only the latest of many groups of desperately sick people who have found hope and consolation on the fringe. This may all be very unsatisfactory from the viewpoint of scientific medicine, but even if the complementary practitioners have nothing more to offer than sympathy and hope, they are clearly exercising a useful function, and one that is valued by the people who consult them.

One other point: in saying that complementary medicine is less likely to recognize limits to its achievements, I don't mean that a herbalist seeing someone with a compound fracture of the leg will offer a tincture of this or that and send the sufferer hobbling on his way. Unless the practitioner is a complete fanatic, he or she will appreciate that some conditions are best dealt with by others. Herbs may encourage the healing process;

but they're not a substitute for having someone else, skilled in setting fractures, first realign the broken ends of the bone.

These are not the only differences between orthodox and complementary medicine, but they are the key ones. And they help to explain why the term 'healer' is no longer one with which most doctors feel comfortable. In the first place, the word is in clear conflict with the 'body technology' component of modern medicine. The surgeon transplanting your kidney stands in relation to you much as the garage mechanic stands in relation to the car when he is changing the oil filter. To describe either as 'healing' seems inappropriate. There is, of course, a difference between the two, but not until the physical task is complete. When the garage mechanic has replaced the oil filter and closed the bonnet, he is unlikely to sit down by the car and speak to it. After an operation, when the surgeon is talking to his patient, examining and dressing the wound, offering comfort and reassurance... these are moments when he *can* be said to be playing the part of a healer. Because the complementary therapist has fewer preoccupations with instrumentation and technological gew-gaws, more of his or her personality, concentration and sympathy is available to the patient. If healing is the therapeutic effect of one person upon another, the complementary practitioner clearly has a greater claim to the title.

None of this, however, explains why doctors find the word healer an embarrassment. I suspect that it has much to do with the science base of their training. One of the tenets of scientific investigation is that the experimenter is not part of the experiment. Although it was Galileo who first demonstrated that cannonballs of unequal weight dropped from the tower of Pisa hit the ground at the same time (many people having believed that the heavier would fall faster), his identity is only of historical interest. If it was the hand of the Pope that had released the balls, the result would have been the same; if you or I did the experiment the outcome would be the same. The result is independent of the observer.

The scientific training that doctors receive tempts them to behave as if the medicine they practise is as independent of them as gravity was of Galileo. The word 'healer', with its faintly mystical connotations seems to run counter to the neat, intellectual purity of the scientific ideal. If men *were* machines, medicine *would* be independent of the doctor, given a certain level of competence, who performed it. But they're not – so it isn't.

Superficially, this distaste for the role of healer seems engagingly self-effacing. It is as if the doctors were striving to avoid personality cults; as if the profession was saying, 'We're not important. It's what we *know* and what we can *do* for you that is all that really counts.' Maybe that is what lies behind it; maybe they really are striving for the higher truth. Somehow, though, I think not. A more likely explanation is that access to science is in itself a form of power – just as access to God has always conferred power on the priests. And the assurance that what really counts in medicine is what is done, not who is doing it, provides an excellent justification for retaining a comfortable degree of detachment from the patients and their troubles.

That doctors recognize the part played by non-material influences in therapy is apparent from their acceptance of placebo factors in treatment and experiment. But one thing that virtually no clinical trials take into account is the possible effect of personality differences between the doctors taking part. Where only one doctor is involved, the importance of his individual characteristics will be minimal, because all patients will be subject to it. But clinical trials nowadays may involve thousands of patients being cared for by many different doctors working in different locations. The committees that devise and regulate such trials draw up elaborate protocols intended to eliminate differences between participating centres and individuals. As long as all the doctors taking part are carrying out the same procedures in the same way, it is assumed that other differences are of no consequence. This may be true. Or the difference may be too small to matter. Either way, there are questions of practicality; there is a limit to the size of a trial that a doctor can run single-handed. In the end, though, it is mischievous but entertaining to speculate that individual personality differences between doctors are ignored in such trials because it helps to maintain the comfortable fiction that they don't matter anyway!

Attitudes to each other

In contrast to the relatively tight, cohesive structure of orthodox medicine, complementary medicine is fragmented to the point of anarchy. So while the doctors have an establishment view of their unorthodox counterparts, it is impossible to say that complementary medicine has any agreed view. To the extent that any organization in Britain can be described as the voice of the establishment in complementary medicine, it would probably be the Council for Complementary and Alternative Medicine (CCAM). This serves as a lobbying body to represent the interests of the major complementary professions. How far some of the smaller and more obscure therapies would feel that its views were also theirs is debatable. Its general stance is one of co-operation with orthodox medicine – which is not surprising because some of its members are themselves doctors.

Some practitioners in a few branches of complementary medicine do not, however, speak with such moderation. Some of them have a positive loathing of mainstream medicine. Its treatment of cancer has often been singled out for excoriating criticism. The three approaches conventionally used – surgery, radiotherapy and drugs – are caricatured and derided as 'cutting', 'burning' and 'poisoning'. More paranoid elements on the fringe seem to believe that mainstream medicine is not only wilfully ignoring alternative methods of treatment, but also engaged in some perverse plot to harm patients. Claims like this do little for the peace of mind of any unfortunate person about to receive one of these treatments.

On the whole, however, the views of complementary practitioners are more benign than this. There is irritation that hospital doctors in particular fail to take more interest in alternatives, puzzlement that orthodox medicine should put so much store by its scientific criteria, envy of the resources lavished (relatively speaking) on orthodox research, delight over the upturn in the fortune of complementary medicine that has come in the past decade or so, and the genuine sorrow born of a belief that so many ways of solving so many illnesses are still being neglected.

The BMA report

One of the biggest setbacks to the relationship between orthodox and complementary medicine was the publication in 1986 of an ill-judged report by the British Medical Association's Board of Science Working Party on Alternative Therapy. The BMA had been stung into commissioning this by its 1982/83 president, the Prince of Wales. The Association's officers were doubtless pleased to have attracted such illustrious patronage, but, like the architects, the doctors have learned that Prince Charles is not always content to act solely as a figurehead. During a speech to the BMA, he urged its members to remember that there is more to medicine than science alone. 'By concentrating on smaller and smaller fragments of the body, modern medicine perhaps loses sight of the patient as a whole being, and by reducing health to a mechanical functioning it is no longer able to deal with the phenomenon of healing.'

The BMA's first mistake was to convene a working party of doctors who, though eminent and accomplished, included no one with particular expertise in complementary medicine. This suggested an unhealthy degree of pre-judgement; certainly it can't have been for want of a suitable doctor with knowledge of the topic.

The working party called for and received written evidence from many bodies and individuals, commissioned the views of one or two experts, mulled the whole lot over, and then issued its report. This began by welcoming the sense of enquiry that had aroused public interest in alternative therapies, but swiftly added that this must be seen as one facet of a wider and less welcome change in society. 'The thesis that we have become a more materialistic, less law-observing, less caring society is perhaps a too sweeping generalization. Yet it is one the city-dweller would recognize.' It went on to identify what it called 'a quite general criticism of governence ... from which orthodox medicine is itself not immune.'

This is breathtakingly arrogant. In effect, while still on page three, the report is already hinting that all this alternative stuff is dangerous nonsense dreamed up by malcontents whose real interest is to find yet another excuse to knock the establishment. If comments like this were to be made at all in the report, a more appropriate place for them would have been in its final summing up. Common sense would suggest that you don't question the motives of those with claims to make until you have at least considered the possibility that their claims may have some validity. Instead, these pages seem to represent the views of men who knew the answers before they had asked the questions and seen the evidence. Hardly an appropriate approach for a Board of *Science*. And hardly in keeping with the working party's own terms of reference, which asked it to 'consider the feasibility and possible methods of assessing the value of alternative therapies, whether used alone or to complement other treatments ...' No call there for careless pseudo-sociological explanations of the new public interest in complementary medicine.

Having meandered through a selection of alternative therapies from acupuncture to radionics, the report's authors offer some general views on the nature of scientific as opposed to complementary medicine. The work and the thinking of doctors, they say, 'are based on scientific method, defining "science" in the strictest sense of the word, namely the systematic observation of natural phenomena for the purpose of discovering laws governing those phenomena.' And elsewhere,

WHO ARE THE HEALERS NOW?

As an integral part of the society in which we live, scientific methodology is generally held to be an acceptable basis on which to set reliable judgements, free from overriding social values and political bias ... Thus, herein lies the first and most important difficulty that orthodox science has with alternative approaches. So many of them do not base their rationale on any theory that is consistent with natural laws as we now understand them ... To medical scientists, the methods and approaches of many alternative therapies seem closely allied to philosophies long since discredited by advancing knowledge.

The report also offers what it regards as the clinching argument: 'The fact is that the steadily developing body of orthodox medical knowledge has led to large, demonstrable and reproducible benefits for mankind, of a scale which cannot be matched by alternative approaches.'

Up to this point in the discussion the logic of the argument is sound, and the preamble to the final section looks equally encouraging: '... some doctors feel uncomfortable when faced by vague somatic complaints which are actually expressions of emotional tensions, and they are happier with physical illness which can be diagnosed and cured.' Who could dispute that? And elsewhere, emphasizing that patients are whole persons with disabilities rather than mere living disease processes the report concedes that, 'To the extent that consideration of alternative therapies draws attention to these features, it has real value ...'

In the end, though, the hint of patronage in the last quote becomes a blast: 'In fairness to the practitioners of alternative medicine, it has to be said that many patients are comforted, and may be "healed", when under their care. It is also possible that among the multiplicity of techniques there are some which are genuinely therapeutic, even beyond any placebo effect.' And then the punch: 'Careful study of this possibility is needed, with a view to bringing beneficial techniques within the safeguards offered by a registered profession' (i.e. medicine).

There is a lot of sound reasoning in the report. But it has two flaws. While it rightly argues for a scientific assessment of therapeutic techniques, it cannot countenance the notion that there might be a place in medicine for methods that science can't easily verify, or that patients want despite its lack of theoretical validity. (This is, admittedly, a difficult issue, and I'll be returning to it.) The other problem with the report is that it wants to maintain medical hegemony: 'Let's find out if aromatherapy really works; if it does, we doctors will take it over and incorporate it into our own practice.' There are several objections to this; for the moment let's say that doctors are ill-suited to taking over many complementary therapies, and some would almost certainly make a mess of them if they tried. I shall be arguing later that what the doctors should be doing is not seeking to take control, but to co-operate.

Other medical views

The BMA report provoked a great deal of criticism, not all of it from complementary practitioners. Indeed, a few years on the report is looking more and more like a rearguard action against a change of heart that was already overtaking some of the BMA's own members, and overturning traditional hostilities.

As with others of its kind, the medical establishment has always been intellectually conservative, jealous of its privileges, and reluctant to concede anything that might diminish its power. One embodiment of the medical establishment in Britain is the General Medical Council, the organization that sets educational standards, maintains a register of qualified practitioners, and organizes the tribunals by which doctors accused of unethical conduct can be judged and sentenced to temporary or even permanent erasure from the medical register. As already pointed out, the profession first sought the right to exclude those of its own who themselves had the effrontery to use unconventional methods. This power was denied them; but the GMC did get the right to strike off any doctor aiding unregistered practitioners, or referring patients to them.

Although this ruling made life more difficult for complemen-

WHO ARE THE HEALERS NOW?

tary practitioners, it didn't prevent the public from consulting them. Among this public were a not inconsiderable number of doctors. The hypocrisy of a regulation that forbade a doctor recommending to one of his or her patients a form of treatment that he or she was receiving finally provoked change. In the early 1970s the GMC ruled that a doctor *could* send someone to a non-medical practitioner provided that the doctor retained overall responsibility. And that, in theory, is how things stand at present.

Evidence that the BMA's working party was out of touch with the views of family doctors, especially younger ones, can be found in a report published in 1983 in the Association's own journal. Dr David Taylor Reilly, then a general practitioner trainee, carried out a survey of fellow trainees attending their annual conference in Scotland. His questionnaire ranged over fifteen therapies from 'the virtually accepted (hypnosis) through the controversial (faith healing) to the esoteric (colour therapy)'.

Dr Reilly found what he describes as a 'striking degree of interest'. Some four out of five wished to train in at least one of the methods on the list (hypnosis was the most popular) and a fifth of them already used at least one of them. More than a third had referred patients for treatment by others using hypnosis, manipulation, homeopathy or acupuncture, and a quarter had themselves received treatment of some sort. By and large the doctors only expressed opinions about those techniques of which they had some knowledge. Dr Reilly did not claim that his findings were representative of the profession at large. A pilot study had already revealed much less interest among junior hospital doctors. But they do seem to signal the emergence of an open-mindedness in general practice that one would never have suspected from reading the BMA working party's report on alternative medicine.

Three years later Drs Richard Wharton and George Lewith of the Centre for the Study of Alternative Therapies in Southampton organized a similar study among GPs in Avon. They found that just over a third had taken some training in a complementary technique, and that an even greater proportion had referred patients for treatment by an unconventional technique. They found a great interest in complementary medicine among GPs, but also a great deal of ignorance and misunderstanding. What they didn't find was evidence of antagonism. And there is good reason to suspect that relations between many individual GPs and complementary practitioners have grown even closer in the years between then and now.

In summary, there exist major differences between orthodox and complementary medicine, both in the methods they use, and in the theories that underpin them. The conventional view that this debars the two groups from co-operating with each other is manifestly untrue. But what little co-operation does exist has usually been the consequence of local initiatives on the part of individual enthusiasts. The question is whether such small scale co-operation could be organized more generally and more widely, and whether patients would benefit as a result. This is an issue I'll return to in the final chapter.

8 Harnessing the Placebo Effect
Its role in orthodox and alternative medicine

At risk of the inevitable injustice to individuals, the attitudes of orthodox and alternative medicine towards the placebo effect can be summarized in a sentence. Orthodox practitioners may know a little or a lot about it, but seldom make an effort to exploit their knowledge; alternative practitioners often know little or nothing about it, but put it to good use – albeit, in many cases, quite unconsciously. First, then, the orthodox camp.

Interest in the placebo effect has been a long time coming and is even now still a largely negative one. As discussed in Chapter 2, medicine's main concern has been not to exploit the placebo effect, but to discount it. Serious consideration of its extent and significance didn't begin until the 1930s – in which decade the handful of doctors who did give it some thought seem to have responded in the same way as almost everyone who comes across the phenomenon for the first time: how can so valuable a thing have been so disregarded? As one author writing in the 1940s pointed out, 'although placebos are scarcely mentioned in the literature, they are administered more than any other group of drugs ... although few doctors admit that they give placebos, there is a placebo ingredient in practically every prescription ... the placebo is a potent agent and its actions can resemble almost any drug.'

Writing in 1960, Dr Arthur Shapiro of New York University

College of Medicine offered several explanations for the belated interest in the phenomenon. Some physicians, he suggested, may find the whole topic embarrassing or even guilt-inducing. He had in mind the use of placebos to treat difficult or demanding patients, or to console those for whom there is no specific remedy. More fancifully Dr Shapiro also suggests that some doctors may be 'threatened by a real or imagined loss of self-esteem and prestige among colleagues and in the community, and by the threat of uncertainty or loss of magical powers'.

I suspect that the truth is simpler than this. By the time that doctors had woken up to the existence of the placebo effect, they had already fallen in love with the powerful and demonstrable benefits of scientific medicine. After centuries of having had nothing to offer except the placebo effect, they had begun to acquire an array of powerful and effective drugs, and a burgeoning technology. They could at last do things to and for patients with predictable and beneficial effects. No wonder that ideas about the innate capacity of the body to heal itself, and the extent to which that capacity might be boosted by rather vague entities such as 'faith' and 'confidence' seemed rather unexciting, rather backward looking. It was as if a man who had relied on using witchcraft and spells to maintain his car in working order had, for the first time, been given a workshop manual and a set of tools. The invention of the double blind controlled trial, while acknowledging the existence of the placebo effect, paradoxically served only to marginalize it as the baseline against which a 'real' treatment could be assessed.

Getting the most out of the placebo effect

The findings of several research studies would appear to offer doctors a number of ways of exploiting the placebo effect. What is known about the significance of pill colour is one of the most obvious, albeit one of the more trivial, examples. The onus in this instance is on the pharmaceutical industry rather than on the doctors. When you recall the vast sums of money that drug companies are prepared to spend on advertising their products, it seems decidedly odd that they show so little interest in anything but the purely pharmacological action of those products. The industry has no scruples about advertisements that rely on non-pharmacological factors to motivate the doctor to prescribe. Yet it seems to make no attempt to use such factors to maximize the benefits that patients get from that drug. One can only surmise that drug companies fear that if they were to be discovered taking too close an interest in the subconscious influences exercised by their products, they would be criticized in much the way they are already for trying to manipulate doctors' prescribing habits.

Where a medicine is likely to be tasted before it's swallowed, flavour, too, must be a consideration. The old saw has it that the nastier the taste, the more good it does. In the light of the placebo effect, and given the general assumption that taking a medicine is not supposed to be a pleasant experience, it is likely that nasty tasting medicines are indeed more effective! Better still is to administer the drug by injection. There are parts of the Third World where patients insist on having their drugs, especially antibiotics, by this means; who can doubt that those who believe that injections are more beneficial do, in fact, obtain more benefit...

Better a professor?

The setting in which the treatment is offered might also turn out to be important. There is evidence that patients taking part in research studies benefit from this knowledge. It seems quite possible that all sorts of other variables could affect the outcome of the treatment: a teaching as opposed to an ordinary district general hospital; a private as opposed to a State institution; a well-maintained health centre as against a rundown lock-up surgery; a senior doctor as opposed to a junior one; one who's entitled 'professor' rather than merely 'doctor'. There is, admittedly, a point at which this starts to become ridiculous: the therapeutic benefits of having a handsome as opposed to an ugly doctor might well represent the sticking point for even the most research-minded clinician! My point in making this *reductio ad absurdum* is simply to demonstrate that placebo effects are ubiquitous.

Cynics have suggested – and not without evidence – that any doctor deploying a new treatment should ensure that as many people as possible receive it at the first opportunity. The very fact that both patient and doctor are aware that a drug is new boosts its placebo potential. But novelty is a diminishing asset. Hence the injunction to treat widely and treat soon! More serious is the ethical question of how far it is legitimate to deceive a patient in the interest of boosting the placebo response.

The most open use of placebos in medicine today is in clinical research on the properties of new drugs. If there is an existing drug for the condition being treated, this will normally be given to the comparison or control group of patients. Any difference between the experimental and the control group of patients is then presumed to arise from specific differences between the two drugs. But where there is no accepted treatment, the control group will usually be given a placebo. The use of such a dummy treatment is generally regarded as ethically acceptable. Although some doctors still debate the point, the current thinking among students of medical ethics is that patients who have agreed to take part in such an experiment should be told that there is a fifty:fifty (or whatever) chance that the pill they get will be, unknown to them, a dummy. The evidence suggests that this knowledge has no adverse effects on the validity of the trial.

Other than in clinical trials, data about doctors' use of placebos is scant. One standard textbook of clinical pharmacology has estimated that as many as 35 to 45 per cent of all prescriptions are for substances incapable of having any effect on the conditions for which they've been prescribed. But this would seem to have more to do with incompetence than with exploitation of the placebo effect. On the other hand, a study of treatments for the common cold found that a surprising 53 per cent of patients were prescribed antibiotics. The common cold is caused by a virus, and viruses do not respond to antibiotics. As it is difficult to believe that any doctor could be unaware of this, the only conclusion to be drawn is that the practitioners concerned (possibly in response to patient pressure, though this is no excuse) were prescribing antibiotics for their placebo value. And it's true that antibiotics *do* have a good placebo value; the very word impresses.

Official placebo

One of the very few official nods to the existence of placebos became apparent on 1 April 1985 when the Government began limiting the number of medicines in certain categories that can be prescribed through the NHS. A couple of thousand antacids, laxatives, minor analgesics, cough and cold remedies, vitamins, inhalations and expectorants were henceforth available only to patients prepared to pay for them. The relatively short 'white' list of permitted products contained only those that were obviously beneficial or value for money in the light of modern pharmacological understanding. There was, however, one anomaly. In the category 'bitters and tonic' two products were permitted: gentian mixture acid, and gentian mixture alkaline.

Given the intentions of the limited list, this is a category that might have been expected to disappear altogether. Bitters, which are among the ingredients of many tonics, are designed to stimulate salivation and appetite. Tonics themselves are designed to pep you up when you feel run down. This notion may retain some popular appeal, but it has little scientific basis. Tonics – of which there have been many – are usually based on some traditional formula, and often contain ingredients that are pharmacologically active. But the idea that panaceas like this will benefit everyone who's feeling below par is unsustainable. So why did they appear in the Government's stripped down, scientifically rational, limited list? The answer – unstated, of course – is obvious. Doctors who felt they had to prescribe *something* for patients who needed no treatment, or whose condition was not suitable for treatment, had to have something innocuous to rely on.

The dilemma for a doctor may be to know what form of words to use when prescribing such a medicine. Several constructions come readily to mind. 'This may help you', does no offence to the truth; placebos *do* help the people who take them. 'In my experience, many patients with a problem similar to yours respond quite well to this medicine', is a more elaborate but similar form of words with much the same advantages and drawbacks.

Sissela Bok, writing in 1974 in *Scientific American*, pointed out that placebos can be harmful to patients – not so much on account of the agent itself as of the manipulation and deception that accompany their prescription.

> Inevitably some patients find out that they have been duped. They may then lose confidence in physicians and in bona fide medication, which they may need in the future. They may even resort on their own to more harmful drugs or other supposed cures. That is a danger associated with all deception: its discovery leads to a failure of trust when trust may be needed. Alternatively, some people who do not discover the deception and are left believing that a placebo remedy works may continue to rely on it under the wrong circumstances. This is particularly true with respect to drugs, such as antibiotics, that are sometimes used for their specific action and sometimes as placebos. Many parents, for example, come to believe they must ask for the prescription of antibiotics every time their child has a fever.

Sissela Bok goes on to concede that there are circumstances in which the prescription of a placebo is without doubt the lesser of two evils. Harm is then most likely to be mitigated by following a number of rules:

1 placebos should be used only after a careful diagnosis;
2 no active placebos should be employed, merely inert ones;
3 no outright lie should be told, and questions should be answered honestly;

4 placebos should never be given to patients who have asked not to receive them;
5 placebos should never be used when other treatment is clearly called for or all possible alternatives have not been weighed.

This is all very reasonable, but one of the relatively few formal studies of the extent to which doctors are not only aware of the placebo effect, but also seek to exploit it came to some disturbing conclusions. Three doctors working at the University of New Mexico asked sixty house officers and a similar number of nurses to complete questionnaires designed to find out how much they understood about the placebo response. They also checked the records of the hospital pharmacy to find out how often placebos were prescribed.

It soon became obvious that most of the doctors surveyed considerably under-estimated the scale of the placebo effect. When asked what proportion of patients might obtain adequate pain relief from a dummy injection administered on the day after an abdominal operation, the doctors' suggested average was 20 per cent (as against the 30–40 per cent figure that has emerged in experimental studies). Nurses put the figure even lower, at about 5 per cent.

Many of the doctors who claimed to know that placebos can relieve post-operative pain in at least some patients still described using a placebo preparation to test if a patient's reported pain was 'real'. They seemed unaware of the contradiction in their logic.

Overall the number of occasions on which placebo preparations were prescribed was very small, about one prescription per doctor per year. Only five of the inpatients treated during the study period received a placebo; but four out of these five had been referred to a psychiatrist on the grounds that they were 'problem' patients.

The American researchers found that the conscious use of placebos fell into several categories, none of which they were entirely happy with. One, already mentioned, was to prove the patient wrong: to find out if his or her claimed pain was genuine. Another was for 'undeserving' patients such as difficult alcoholics: individuals who were not felt to merit the gift of a proper, pharmacologically active drug. Wondering what can be done to prevent these misuses of the placebo effect, the researchers point out that few of the nurses or doctors in their survey had had any formal instruction about placebos. Unfortunately, knowledge is not the only key; some of the house officers who took part in the study used placebos in a way that their own understanding should have told them was futile. This paradoxical state of affairs only begins to make sense when it is realized that most placebos were prescribed in circumstances of severe hostility between staff and patients. The anxiety so generated seems to have interfered with rational judgement.

Doctor placebo

The doctor is on much safer territory when trying to exploit one other aspect of his potential for inducing a placebo effect: himself. In Chapter 1 I quoted the psychiatrist Dr Michael Balint as having pointed out that the most frequently used drug in general practice is the doctor himself. In the same article he goes on to regret that this important drug has, as yet, no pharmacology.

No textbook advises the doctor as to the dosage in which he should prescribe himself, in what form, and how frequently. Nor is there any literature on the hazards of this kind of medication, on the allergic responses encountered, or on the undesirable side effects. The reassuring statement is often made that experience and common sense will help the doctor to acquire the necessary skill in prescribing himself. But this is very different from the very careful and detailed instructions with which every new drug is nowadays introduced into general practice.

Such elementary considerations have yet to impress themselves on some doctors. The consultant who prefers to talk to his juniors than talk to his patients is familiar to anyone who has spent time in hospital; likewise the habit of talking about the patient as if he or she is an inanimate object. There are rude doctors and cold doctors; there are doctors who offer no greeting when you enter the surgery; doctors who spend the entire consultation scribbling in the notes or on the prescription pad, and shun anything resembling eye contact; there are doctors who won't listen, doctors who patronize or who seem uninterested, and doctors who can't get their patients out of the surgery fast enough. All these elementary faults in attitude and behaviour serve to diminish the placebo effect of the doctor, serve to make him or her a less effective healer.

One particularly striking example of the doctor as a placebo is to be found in the person of the late William Sargent, a psychiatrist who was influential in the development of his branch of medicine. As a young doctor, he was appalled by what he saw of life inside the mental hospitals – the only refuge for anyone severely afflicted with major psychiatric illnesses such as schizophrenia. This experience fuelled his determination to improve psychiatry – which was then limited to little more than certifying lunatics, and acting as their custodians. William Sargent's achievement was to champion the then relatively new idea that mental illness might have an organic cause, and be suitable for treatment by physical methods, in particular, drugs. The breakthrough in this respect was the discovery of the phenothiazines. The best known of these, chlorpromazine (Largactil), was developed in 1951. Major tranquillizers of this kind control manic patients without impairing their consciousness so that they become socially more compliant. They relieve many of the symptoms of schizophrenia, allowing patients whose behaviour had previously kept them in hospital to live in the community. Despite the poor reputation of drugs like this (the 'chemical cosh'), without them it is inconceivable that the mental hospitals of today would be as empty as they have become.

Because William Sargent was so committed to the treatment of mental illness by physical methods, he was inclined to regard psychotherapy – indeed all talking treatments – as irrelevant. He took the view that if you didn't rely on talking to patients to cure their measles or their inflamed appendices, why should you when dealing with their abnormally functioning brains? But while Sargent preached that what really counted were the treatments themselves, the fact was that many patients would seek help from him in particular, and sometimes respond to his treatment when those of others had failed. It wasn't because his pills were better or stronger than those of other doctors; it was his exceptionally forceful personality they were responding to. In this respect William Sargent was a living contradiction of his own beliefs that mental illness was solely an organic disorder that happened to manifest itself in a non-organic manner. Either way he was a classic example of the doctor as placebo.

Medical training

It is now generally realized that there is value in training doctors not only to be good body technicians, but also to relate to their patients as people. The Todd report on medical education tried to foster this change when it was published twenty years ago. If the training of medical students has still not changed as much as some people would like, the hurdles are now as much to do with the over-crowding of the curriculum as with any reluctance on the part of medical schools to introduce change. Several schools have adopted one particular innovation in training: the use of actors as patients on whom students can test their skills without causing distress to real patients. As one tutor at Leicester University Medical School put it to a group of students, none of whom were eager to volunteer for the hot seat in an exercise designed to test their skill in breaking bad news, 'This is the only time in your lives you'll have the opportunity to make a mess of telling someone they've got multiple sclerosis.'

To some doctors, of course, empathy with patients comes naturally; to others it is a struggle. But there is no one, good or bad at talking and listening, whose performance can't be improved by thinking about the task, and perhaps following a few simple guidelines. Of course, medical schools that give a place to this kind of teaching do so on the grounds that doctors should behave humanely, not because they're trying to boost the doctor's placebo effect. This outcome is incidental.

Thinking about the placebo effect does raise one intriguing question about the new orthodoxy in the relationships between doctors and patients. In the past these were almost wholly authoritarian: the doctor told the patient what he or she should do, and the patient did it. Times change and this began to seem anachronistic. Doctors nowadays are supposed to encourage patients to play a part in reaching decisions; the doctor lays various treatment options before the patients who must make up their own minds. This way of doing things may still be honoured as much in the breach as the acceptance; but it is certainly how progressive doctors try to behave. The question is this: how far is the doctor's authority responsible for inducing the placebo effect? And if it *is* playing a part, has the striving for more equality in doctor–patient relationships undermined it? Advocates of the new orthodoxy would no doubt argue that it is a case of swings and roundabouts; that whatever placebo effect may have been lost in the decline of authority has been more than made up for in the feelings of confidence that come when people behave more autonomously. The truth of the matter is that what has been lost and what gained must depend on the personality and outlook of each individual patient. In this respect there are probably winners *and* losers.

Placebos: the alternative view

Some doctors, pressed to say what they really think, would argue that much of complementary medicine is one huge and elaborate exploitation of the placebo effect. Those who know the history of their own profession will be aware of the point made several times earlier in this book: that, until quite recently, most of the treatments offered by most practitioners – no matter whether or not they called themselves doctors – had few if any useful specific effects. Just as previous generations of quacks and charlatans peddled snake oil, and got away with it on account of the placebo effect, so too do the fringe practitioners of today.

Strip away the vested interest and arrogance that infected the BMA's forlorn attempt to tackle this issue, and you find a powerful case to be answered by the complementary fraternity. The recurring difficulty in any consideration of complementary medicine is that having no coherent identity other than its nonorthodoxy, it has no single view on such matters. Its practitioners range from people with higher degrees in medicine through to those who have learnt their stuff by taking a six-week correspondence course. So to say that complementary practitioners think this or that is virtually impossible.

The chief argument for viewing complementary medicine as reliant on the placebo effect is the absence of evidence that this is not the case. When placebo responses of the order of 30 per cent can be achieved simply by giving someone a dummy pill, those who make claims for the specific benefits of a remedy clearly have to take on the burden of proof. The presumption must be that therapeutic success, until proved otherwise, is a consequence of the placebo effect. This is a harsh discipline – but no harsher than scientific medicine has learned to apply to its own efforts. Anyone claiming that such and such a treatment is effective in x per cent of cases should be able to answer two questions: How has the improvement been assessed? and With whom have the treated patients been compared? Unless those questions can be answered, sceptics have every right to suspect that the improvement may be a consequence of spontaneous remission (most things *do* get better by themselves) aided by the placebo effect.

By this test, a great many branches of complementary medicine do not do well. Some make no effort at all to substantiate their claims. Others have professional journals in which they give details of patients' case histories, and describe how they have responded to certain treatments. Such reports may offer useful pointers; but they have little to do with proof. Even reports of success in treating a large number of similar cases by similar means do little to demonstrate efficacy if there is no control group of patients with whom to make comparisons. But then such journals, and the reports they carry, are really meant only for the committed, for believers.

Of course, orthodox medical journals also carry case reports. In the case of, say, penicillin it is no longer necessary to publish controlled trials of its effectiveness; these were done long ago and we know what it does and under what circumstances. Nowadays, a single case history in which penicillin given to a particular patient provoked an unusual response *would* be of interest. Case histories of this kind are not unlike those you may find in unorthodox medical journals. The difference is that in the unorthodox case the groundwork of proof has never been attempted.

When you consider the painfully exacting methods and the lifetimes of laborious work by which science analyses the nature of disease, devises treatments, and then tests them, it's hardly surprising that doctors become testy when confronted with practitioners who apparently 'know', without any discernible effort, that this disease is caused by the patient's internal constitution being out of balance, and that that illness is attributable to a weakness in his energy flow. You don't have to be utterly under the spell of the puritan work ethic to believe that really useful knowledge about the world is seldom acquired without effort, and that understandings derived from personal revelation are seldom worth as much as those acquired through empirical investigation. Science and scientific medicine are suffused with a spirit of scepticism; 'prove it' is the ever-present challenge. By comparison, alternative medicine is a very cosy place. Instead of scepticism, the prevailing ethos is one that often veers dangerously close to credulity. In this all-embracing tranquillity, the challenge to 'prove it' would be as out of keeping as obscene language at a royal garden party. To those accustomed to the brisk intellectual debate of science, the fringe seems a soft and woolly thing.

Equally disconcerting are the plethora of theories that underpin complementary medicine. Concepts such as 'internal energy flow' mean nothing at all to science. These energies usually have no objective manifestation (other than the symptoms they are said to cause), and can't be measured by orthodox techniques. They have to be taken on trust, something totally at odds with the expectations and assumptions of science. To take an example from modern physics, recall the brouhaha over the existence or otherwise of cold fusion. Scientists Martin Fleischmann and Stanley Pons claimed to have found a way of persuading the energy-generating process of the Sun to take place at room temperature. The discovery had vast theoretical and practical implications, and aroused great interest among physicists around the world. But no one assumed that because the two scientists were men with good professional reputations their claims should be taken on trust. As things have turned out, this was fortunate.

Sceptics have often claimed – with reason – that it would be quite easy to invent a completely bogus therapy, and then make a living out of it. Glancing through a list of what is currently available, the main problem would seem to be finding something that someone isn't already doing.

Absence of proof

When challenged about the absence of proof that they're doing anything other than relying on the placebo effect, complementary practitioners offer several explanations – some more persuasive than others. The most fundamental objection is that conventional scientific research methods are inappropriate for investigating unconventional treatments. Superficially this argument is persuasive; the double blind controlled trial beloved of medical researchers relies on identifying a single variable – usually the drug being tested – and discounting all other factors by keeping them the same for all subjects. Complementary practitioners argue that their techniques cannot be fitted into such a framework; they choose the treatment not only according to the nature of the illness, but also the nature of the person. Moreover they may change the treatment from time to time. And to discount the relationship between the practitioner and the patient makes a nonsense of the assessment because this relationship is a part of the therapy.

The objection is legitimate; but this simply means that the techniques of validation have to be adapted. This has indeed been done, notably in a Medical Research Council study of chiropractic for low back pain. The chiropractors are one group of complementary practitioners who have been keen to see their methods scrutinized. In collaboration with them, the MRC devised a mutually acceptable methodology. In essence, the organizers of the trial identified patients with low back pain for whom chiropractic should be a suitable form of treatment. These patients were then allocated at random to a chiropractor, or to their local hospital. In both cases they then received whatever treatment the staff looking after them judged most appropriate. In other words, this trial assessed entire chiropractic and conventional medical treatment packages. The results, as it turned out, tended to favour chiropractic.

The trial did not pass without controversy. Critics pointed to its weaknesses; for example, it revealed nothing of which elements of the chiropractors' therapies might be valuable, and which unhelpful. Overall, though, it showed that the task of evaluating complementary medicine on its own terms, and by methods that are scientifically respectable is not impossible.

This wasn't in fact the first attempt to do something of the kind. As mentioned earlier, in the 1970s doctors in Glasgow compared the relative benefits of homeopathic remedies, aspirin and a placebo to patients suffering from rheumatoid arthritis. Conventional doctors administered the aspirin, homeopathically trained doctors the homeopathic remedies, and the results were judged by independent assessors. Both actively treated groups did better than those who received only a placebo. Doctors and patients alike agreed that there wasn't much to choose between the two active remedies as far as the progress of the disease was concerned. There was, however, one important difference: the homeopathic remedies produced fewer side effects.

A more severe barrier to research is the indifference of many of the complementary practitioners themselves. Those utterly convinced of the efficacy of what they are doing see experiments designed to find out if it really works as being at best irrelevant, at worst (if it would involve depriving some patients of treatment) unethical. Let those who disbelieve do the studies, is their attitude. The snag is that those who disbelieve – generally orthodox physicians – have little inclination to do so; any time that they have available for research they usually wish to devote to topics that they view as potentially more fruitful. The same kind of arguments surface over the matter of funding: orthodox grant-giving bodies have little enthusiasm for funding research into unorthodox techniques when they haven't enough to implement their own agendas; and the complementary practitioners themselves plead lack of resources. This last is sometimes used to disguise a lack of will. Some practitioners with little scientific training just cannot comprehend the zeal for questioning and analysis that is so central to scientific medicine. Such individuals will respond to any challenge about the validity of their methods by pointing to the satisfied patients as evidence. In this respect they are behaving like all previous generations of healers. The difference is that such obduracy is no longer acceptable in an age that has learnt about the placebo effect, and has acquired the tools and the insight to take a more critical view of matters. A reluctance to undertake self-scrutiny invites suspicion that it is born of nervousness about the findings. The only way to counter that charge is, of course, to do the research.

So to what extent are complementary practitioners aware of the placebo effect? The answer must be that no one knows. Those who come to the field from within orthodox medicine certainly know about it. Dr Anthony Campbell of the Royal London Homeopathic Hospital, author of a thoughtful and thought-provoking book on homeopathy, tackles the question of placebos head on:

HARNESSING THE PLACEBO EFFECT

The fact is that almost any kind of treatment you care to think of will appear to work at least some of the time ... For many patients the mere fact of receiving treatment – any treatment, even coloured water – will be beneficial ... Thus in trying to assess the efficacy of any form of treatment the question we have to ask is not *whether* spontaneous recovery, the placebo effect, and so on play a part – there is no doubt they do – but rather *how big* a part they play. In other words, does the treatment do something over and above what would be expected to happen if the patient received either no treatment or a placebo?

It would be reassuring to find a passage such as this in more books on alternative medicine. A skim through the indexes of the collection on my own shelves revealed that references of any kind to placebos or the placebo effect are something of a rarity. Few of these books offer the reader even the slightest hint that there might be questions to be asked about how and why the methods they describe actually work.

In the light of all these considerations, it is clear that the question of how much of the benefit of complementary medicine is attributable to the placebo effect cannot be answered. Viewed through the eyes of an orthodox scientist it is possible to combine the few fragments of evidence that are available with some informed guesswork. For example, any technique that involves relaxation – and many do – is almost certainly producing more than a placebo response. Typical of the evidence that can be cited here is the work of London GP Dr Chandra Patel. She has organized several studies of non-pharmacological methods of managing raised blood pressure, including relaxation. It is clear from published work that relaxation can reduce blood pressure in the short term. However, as she herself points out, many of these experiments have involved highly motivated volunteers who have received one-to-one training of an intensity that would be impracticable for wider use. To put relaxation to a more realistic test, she invited men and women identified as having high blood pressure in an industrial screening programme to attend eight group-training sessions, held at weekly intervals, in deep muscle relaxation, breath control, meditation and stress management. Four years later, those workers who had been taught how to relax were still showing the benefits by comparison with a similar group who had been given only health education advice.

The trial that demonstrated the beneficial effects of chiropractic has already been referred to. So too have the encouraging findings of the study of homeopathy in the treatment of rheumatoid arthritis. One reviewer who scoured the literature in search of controlled trials of homeopathy managed to identify more than a hundred. Their quality varied greatly; but on balance they tended to confirm that homeopathic remedies could be effective.

Acupuncture is a technique with results for which there is certainly persuasive evidence. An American study published in 1980 reported that acupuncture for low back pain had produced an 83 per cent success rate; only 31 per cent of a comparable untreated group had shown any improvement. In this, as in many studies of acupuncture, the weakness lies in the adequacy of the control group of patients. Participants may not be able to detect a dummy pill; but it is abundantly clear to them whether or not someone is inserting a needle! The difference in improvement between the two groups could therefore be the placebo effect of knowing that the acupuncture had been given. One ingenious way round the problem is to devise a piece of bogus apparatus sufficiently impressive to induce a placebo effect of its own. One acupuncturist, assessing its value in back pain, did just this; he wired half of his patients to a six-foot tall box that did nothing, but was covered in flashing lights and dials and made a whirring noise. His patients showed a placebo-induced lessening of their pain. But patients who had had acupuncture showed more improvement.

Another inventive way of ensuring that patients were denied the knowledge of whether or not they had received acupuncture was used by a Danish research group. Their interest was in post-operative pain – so they were able to perform the acupuncture (or not) before the patients had recovered from the anaesthetic. In this experiment, the group who had received acupuncture required only half the pain-killing drugs needed by the un-needled patients.

The most obvious way of testing the benefits of acupuncture is to compare it with a sham procedure in which the needles are inserted at points not regarded as relevant to the condition being treated. Ethically speaking this has the drawback of being an invasive procedure that is not performed for the patient's benefit. Several researchers have none the less overcome any scruples they may have felt about using such a method. In this way, acupuncture has been shown to relieve pains in the back and shoulders and the face, and the pain of rheumatoid arthritis in the knee. It was less successful in treating a group of people with chronic back pain. Similar use of a sham control group has shown acupuncture to be able to overcome the symptoms of asthma, and to quell the nausea associated with pregnancy and with chemotherapy.

The case in favour of aromatherapy – the use of highly-scented essential oils, often massaged into the skin – is rather more equivocal. The scientific evidence of benefit is minimal. In so far as their application involves massage, some specific action on the body seems quite plausible. And the enjoyment to be had from any pleasant odour no doubt makes its contribution to well-being in the way that all pleasurable experiences may be assumed to do. But the claims of aromatherapists are more specific than this: oil of lavender will be recommended for this condition, oil of rosemary for that. It is conceivable that when these oils penetrate the skin they do have specific, pharmacological effects. It is also conceivable (just) that the differing emotional sensations induced by inhaling different odours could have various specific consequences. But the biologist will emphasize that what is conceivable is not necessarily what is probable, let alone what actually happens. The jury is still out on the question of how far aromatherapists can go beyond a placebo effect. So it is good to know that the International Federation of Aromatherapists has begun to show an interest in research.

Radionics lies in a different category again. It relies on forces that make no claims to be anything other than paranormal. The theory is based on the alleged existence of various forces and energy fields, some at least of which can't be detected or measured by orthodox scientific instruments. Diagnosis does not have to be conducted in the presence of the patient; a sample of bodily material, typically a lock of hair, is sufficient. This 'witness' is placed on a metal plate mounted upon an instrument bearing an array of calibrated dials. The operator tunes his mind to the subject who provided the witness, and then twiddles the knobs until he can divine the nature and intensity of the energy disturbance that underlies the patient's suffering. Treatment is also conducted in this manner: at long range and without the presence – or, in some cases, the knowledge – of the fortunate recipient. The aim of the practitioner is to 'open up the channels and allow the life force to flow freely', thereby allowing the body to heal itself. There are various versions of radionics and a number of different pieces of gadgetry.

None of this makes even the slightest sense to orthodox physics. But practitioners have little trouble in finding satisfied clients and speak with pride of their therapeutic triumphs. The placebo effect is not a concept mentioned in any of the radionics manuals I have looked through. Apart from the all-too-successful efforts of amateur tricksters who send in cat hairs or chicken blood as witnesses in an attempt to fool radionics practitioners, there seem to have been no studies designed to validate this most improbable technique. So what to make of it? I can only say that if I had to devise a new but entirely bogus system of healing that would impress potential clients with its fancy instrumentation and its mystical theory, I imagine I would come up with something not unlike radionics.

Healing occupies a particularly interesting place in any consideration of the placebo effect. Various interpretations of its undoubted benefits are possible. Those of a religious persuasion may argue that it represents divine intervention, a view that falls outside the ambit of science. A second interpretation, and the one favoured by many healers themselves, is that what they are doing is acting as a channel by which therapeutic energy from some external source or from the healer is transmitted to the patient. Attempts to identify or measure this energy by the standard methods of physics have been unsuccessful. The third interpretation is that healing represents the purest form of the placebo effect. Healers rely on nothing but themselves, some not even touching the individuals they are trying to help.

Although no one has reported a proper, controlled trial of healing, a number of claims have been made concerning its power to influence events in the laboratory. An American nun, Sister Justa Smith, carried out experiments in which she claimed to be able to use her healing powers to boost an enzyme reaction taking place in a sealed test tube. Whether these and many other such experiments would stand up to detailed scrutiny must remain a matter of speculation. It has to be said that the record of research into all forms of parascience is peppered with instances of inadequate experimental method, if not of deliberate deception.

Complementary medicine comprises scores of different techniques, and the handful so briefly reviewed here have been chosen simply to illustrate that some assuredly do have a specific physiological effect, some almost certainly don't, and some just might. In other words, generalization is impossible. As with any form of therapy, all benefit from the placebo effect. Whether they achieve more than this depends on the therapy; as far as most of them are concerned, this question has to remain open. It must not be forgotten that all the properly controlled trials of complementary medicine that have ever been done probably wouldn't fill more than a year or two's issues of any one of the world's hundreds of conventional medical journals, most of which publish the results of controlled trials, month in month out.

What is apparent is that many complementary techniques, and the circumstances in which they're used, produce a powerful placebo action. The practitioners don't set out to achieve this effect; it is simply a by-product of their firm and entirely correct belief that their relationships to their patients are an important part of the treatment they have to offer. The chiropractors, for example, are exceptionally thorough in training their students in the importance of communicating with their patients; the degree course offered by the Anglo-European College of Chiropractic in Bournemouth includes lectures on psychology that would do merit to any orthodox medical training.

It is important that studies of complementary techniques continue, with the aim of finding out which, if any, of their elements do have specific physiological or pharmacological effects. But so long as the practitioners are sincere about what they're doing and do not deceive their patients, and so long as no one has coerced the patients into this form of therapy, perhaps it doesn't matter too much if some at least of the techniques of alternative medicine are 'only' placebos. The practical implications and possible consequences of this thought will be explored in the final chapter.

9 Mainstream Meets the Fringe

Experiments in co-operation between orthodox and complementary medicine

Many doctors continue to believe that they can best serve their patients by operating primarily as what I have called 'body technicians'. They accept that their work (especially in the case of GPs), of its nature, demands occasional and unavoidable (but preferably brief and not too frequent) diversions into marriage guidance, bereavement counselling and other forms of social support; but they view these matters as secondary to medicine's main purpose.

This body technician role is, indisputably, a vital ingredient of medicine: arguably *the* vital ingredient. But if a study of the placebo effect reveals anything, it is that there's more to practising good medicine than just applying a knowledge of anatomy, physiology and pharmacology. Other factors enter the equation, including the patients' beliefs and perceptions about themselves and their illnesses, and their relationships with their doctors. All good practitioners try to take account of these things, and adjust their actions accordingly. But a handful of GPs, despite having an impeccably orthodox training, go much further than this. They recognize that an increasing number of people are voting with their feet, and seeking out the help of complementary practitioners; they are aware that unorthodox medicine does try to meet those more subtle needs – psychological and even, dare one say it, spiritual – to which orthodox medicine pays no formal regard. Other doctors who are part of this movement have a simpler motive: they think that certain complementary techniques can achieve what orthodox medicine can't, or can do so in a way that is more acceptable to patients. Some use these techniques – homeopathy, acupuncture or whatever – themselves; others work in collaboration with non-medical therapists to whom they refer their patients.

Many of these practitioners would like to run a regular NHS practice in which complementary medicine could be fully integrated. Under the present contractual arrangements between GPs and the National Health Service this is virtually impossible unless the doctors concerned are prepared to sacrifice a substantial part of their own incomes, or they have access to outside funding. Doctors who use complementary techniques argue that many of their interventions are cheaper than those of orthodox medicine, and that in the long run they save the NHS money. Some of these doctors certainly have lower drug bills through, for example, using relaxation instead of anti-hypertensives to deal with high blood pressure. But the true cost-benefit is unknown; and, for the present, even if they could prove they were saving NHS money in other areas, there is no mechanism by which they could claim such savings and use them to run their own practices – NHS accounting doesn't allow for this. Nor is the NHS permitted to employ unregistered practitioners. Hence the two set ups that are actually found in general practice: doctors who, as already mentioned, make a limited use of these techniques themselves; and doctors who perhaps let a room in the same building to one or more complementary practitioners who then use this as a base for their own private practices.

One of Britain's few regular NHS general practices to combine orthodox with complementary medicine, and make no charge to patients for using the latter, is the Marylebone Health Centre in London. Up to a fifth of consultations are with one of the centre's non-medically qualified complementary practitioners, who include an osteopath, a herbalist and a homeopath. In addition, several of the doctors who work there themselves use techniques such as acupuncture or homeopathy. The centre was only able to establish itself because of the support it received from a charity, the Wates Foundation. It can also call on a certain amount of funding from its own charitable trust.

It is surely some indication of the difficulty of setting up an enterprise like the Marylebone Health Centre that, despite the publicity, despite the interest it has aroused, and despite the admiration, it has so few imitators. One other group that *has* managed to get something going is based at Sydenham in South London. The GPs there collaborate with an osteopath and an acupuncturist. Their services are free to patients but, once again, the running costs are met not only by the NHS but also by a charitable foundation.

What follows are brief accounts of three other, very different projects. The first – the closest to the Marylebone model – is an attempt at complete integration of orthodox and complementary medicine. The second shows how complementary medicine can operate within the context of an NHS community clinic. The third illustrates that single individuals, given the motivation, can bring complementary techniques into an orthodox medical setting. All three demonstrate that the two camps *can* work together – if the will is there.

The Blackthorn Trust

In the early 1980s GP Dr David McGavin, then working in Bristol, was nursing a dream of being able to run his own practice in his own way: in particular, to make more use of homeopathy and the other unconventional methods to which he was attracted. The chance came when he became a partner in a Maidstone practice with two other GPs, close to retirement, who were willing to tolerate his eccentric ideas. Dr McGavin claims not to believe in master plans, so it is unlikely that when he first went to the town he'd have guessed that by the beginning of the 1990s he would have founded a medical charity that is pioneering the development of a new element in general practice, and has raised sufficient money to design and build a bigger health centre.

Dr McGavin takes his inspiration from the Austrian scientist and philosopher Rudolf Steiner who died in 1925. Steiner wrote of the value of creativity in helping people to mobilize the resources latent within them, and to restore a lost balance to mind, body and spirit. Like many doctors, David McGavin was aware that medicine as conventionally practised is apt to run out of things to offer when dealing with certain categories of patient. These are people with disorders such as multiple sclerosis for which medicine has no specific treatment; there are chronic illnesses such as Parkinson's disease and rheumatoid arthritis in which the symptoms can be eased, but neither eliminated nor prevented from progressing; and there are large numbers of patients with psychiatric disturbances such as anxiety and depression, which may resist all effort to treat them by standard methods. Most often, patients in this predicament will turn to families, friends or fellow sufferers; seldom can they expect further help from the doctors.

Many GPs, aware that they themselves have nothing more to offer in these circumstances, feel frustrated. And so did David McGavin until he began to work with non-medical therapists who *could* do something for these patients. The Blackthorn Trust has made it possible for him to refer his patients, and those of other local doctors, to therapists who specialize in art, in music, and in a form of movement called eurhythmy. To begin with Dr McGavin spends up to an hour talking to each patient, getting to know them, and exploring their problems in detail. Only then will he pass them on to whichever therapist he judges most likely to be able to help.

On first hearing of this arrangement many people – including some of the patients – are prompted to wonder what relevance, except in a very general sense, art or music can have to someone with a chronic illness. And if these things are indeed relevant, why not just join an evening class? As Dr McGavin explains, these sessions are not designed simply as an entertainment or even an education. Art therapy, for example, is not about how best to draw a bird or paint a tree; and you don't need any skills with the brush. Rather it is about colour: thinking about it, choosing it, relating to it and applying it to the paper, though not necessarily in any representational form.

An example from music therapy can best illustrate the principles that underlie the work. One of the instruments used in the music therapy sessions is the gong. These come in many sizes – from J. Arthur Rank Pictures size down to instruments just a few inches across. Dr McGavin quotes the example of a successful businessman who has had three heart attacks and can't cope with the premature retirement that his health has thrust upon him, and the agoraphobic housewife whose fear of engagement with life is as threatening to her as the businessman's loss of it is to him. In a group session, the therapist might give the large gong to the housewife, and the small one to the businessman. In playing these instruments, he would recognize that small but distinct contributions are as valuable as big and loud ones; she would gain the confidence that comes of making those big and loud sounds.

This example is necessarily simplistic; indeed, it sounds trite. But it has to be said that watching some of these therapy sessions in action is to witness something surprisingly moving. In one music therapy session I went to see, the instruments were hand lyres, flutes and small tubular bells. The half dozen patients involved arranged themselves in a loose semi-circle. Each in turn, from one end of the semi-circle to the other, played a single cord so that the sound seemed to whirl back and forth. As the participants played their instruments they swayed slowly, and quite unselfconsciously, in time with the music. Anyone stumbling across this group activity, and knowing nothing of its purpose, would have been mystified. Indeed, there is an amiable dottiness about the whole enterprise. But it works; an independent survey of its benefits gave it the thumbs up, and local health authorities are now backing the work.

PLEASING THE PATIENT

The patients themselves are enthusiastic – though not all find it easy to define exactly what they get out of it. The Trust also employs a counsellor who talks individually to patients, and leads group discussions. It is not too difficult to see how this might benefit patients. One man, a chronic depressive who has failed for years to respond to conventional psychiatric help, finds relief in an hour of singing on a Monday morning. He can't really say why – except that he is recovering some of his lost confidence, and finding a relief from his depression that he had never experienced during years of formal psychiatric help. Another patient, a woman who has had surgery for a tumour of the colon, which has now spread to her liver, is receiving art therapy. She talks of using pale pinks and blues to paint pictures of the sea and the sky. She says it relaxes her, takes her mind off her problems, and 'helps her emotionally'. Again, very vague – but for her a turning point.

Some of the benefit must come through the non-specific effect of meeting other people with difficulties, exchanging ideas and, by definition, overcoming the social isolation that afflicts many of them. For some reason, these people are finding inner resources that previously they had been unable to tap.

Not just for the middle class

The central economic fact about complementary medicine – that most of it has to be paid for – is no doubt one of the main reasons why it is used disproportionately by the middle class. Whether cash is the sole explanation remains a matter of speculation. But, as it happens, one of the few attempts to set up a community-based complementary medical clinic is located in one of the poorest, most deprived parts of London's East End. It is managed by the Hoxton Health Group, itself comprising local people who are trying to arrange local health care in ways that suit their needs than those of the system.

The idea came from a local community development worker who happened to be a part-time acupuncturist. She recognized that people living in areas like Hoxton, Shoreditch and Bethnal Green – often people with the greatest health and social problems – tend to get the least out of the NHS. She wondered if complementary medicine might meet at least some of their needs rather more successfully than the NHS. It was her good fortune that someone working for the local health authority turned out to be equally enthusiastic. Money from the Government's inner city partnership scheme was used to set up and run the clinic. Its annual running cost in 1991 was about £70,000.

The clinic operates for sixty hours a week and offers a variety of techniques, including relaxation, osteopathy, chiropractic, herbalism, acupuncture, massage and T'ai-chi. In the early days, the practitioners were volunteers; now they are paid, albeit modestly. The patients are restricted to local people aged 55 and over who are members of the Hoxton Health Group. The aim is to focus the help offered by the clinic on those whose needs are the greatest.

Although some patients are referred to the clinic by their GPs, there are still many self-referrals, and most people who hear about the clinic do so by word of mouth. Relationships with the local GPs are good. The commonest reasons for attendance are arthritic problems of various kinds. Stress, anxiety and tension are also well-represented. The patients themselves are enthusiastic, valuing the time they get with the practitioners. As with other users of the NHS, time in the consulting room is something to which they're unaccustomed.

Sweet smells

Liz (not her real name) is an aromatherapist. For the past four years she's been working with patients who are HIV positive, and with those who have full blown AIDS.

The International Federation of Aromatherapists has a programme that it calls Aromatherapy in Care that is designed to encourage its members to work in NHS hospitals and clinics, mostly on a voluntary basis. Liz was particularly touched by the plight of AIDS patients, and felt she had something to offer. Without any great expectations of acceptance she wrote to one of the senior physicians at a hospital dealing with many AIDS patients. He invited her to see him. He admitted that he knew nothing about aromatherapy, but said he was interested in anything that might improve the quality of life of people for whom he could offer no prospect of a cure. He promised to discuss it with his nursing and medical colleagues (who approved) and subsequently with the patients (who were enthusiastic). Liz began working voluntarily one evening a week.

In the early days the hospital directed her to the patients who were most stressed by their condition. They also, she says, kept a very close eye on what she was doing! She likes to spend about an hour and a half with each patient, preferably somewhere quiet and without too many interruptions. With a new patient she spends the first twenty minutes or so simply talking and listening: getting to know that person, to find out as much as she can about the illness, and how he or she feels about it. Aromatherapy in this country consists of massage in association with one or more of some 250 essential oils. Like other therapists, Liz tries to match the oil she uses to the particular condition and needs of the patient. She admits that the choice is at least partly instinctive. She massages patients all over their bodies, sometimes talking to them while she does it, but more often in silence. One of the aims is, after all, to induce a state of relaxation that patients find it otherwise difficult to attain.

Liz repeats the sessions weekly; the first is not always very satisfactory; patients tend to be too conscious of what's happening to relax fully. In subsequent sessions the benefits begin to emerge. Sleep comes more swiftly, and some patients report that it eases their symptoms, including pain.

Thus far the experiment seems to have been a success. There was a small amount of antagonism from medical staff at the beginning; but this has faded away. The only remaining and very occasional problem is with nursing staff – one or two of whom, according to Liz, become jealous of the close relationship she sometimes builds up with long-term patients. The luxury of spending an hour and a half with a single patient is not one given to most nurses in the NHS. Thus far the patients have, without exception, approved of aromatherapy.

Liz's voluntary arrangement – one evening a week at each of two hospitals – continued for the best part of three years. Now she's working four-and-a-half days with AIDS patients, virtually full time. But she still isn't paid by the NHS. Instead she receives a variety of grants and donations from various charities and hospital leagues of friends. Hardly a satisfactory state of affairs for a therapy that seems to have demonstrated its worth.

10 To Please the Patient

A new relationship between orthodox and complementary medicine

Doctor to patient: *Well, Mrs Jones, as I remember it, you've been taking the anti-inflammatory drugs for that arthritis in your knee for, what is it? three years now. You say it's not as stiff as it used to be, which is splendid, and it's really only the occasional bit of pain that is giving you a problem. So I suggest we try you on a course of acupuncture, and find out if you can get by without the drugs. I know you're a bit nervous about the idea of acupuncture, but it really doesn't hurt at all. And we have our own acupuncture clinic every Tuesday afternoon here at the health centre now. So ask the receptionist to make you an appointment, and you can at least have a chat with the acupuncturist. He'll explain it all to you, and I'm sure he'll be able to set your mind at rest.*

Now the other problem, the feelings of anxiety you keep on having. Looking through your notes I see you gave our relaxation class a try, but it didn't make a great deal of difference. The Valium does seem to have helped, but it's not a good idea to use these for more than a few weeks, so now you're feeling a bit calmer I suggest we start running them down, and try something else. A colleague of mine in that new practice along the High Street has just started a weekly aromatherapy clinic. I've no experience of aromatherapy myself, but he tells me that some of the patients in his last practice found it very helpful. So, if you like, I'll give him a ring and see if we can fix something up...

This is not a conversation you'd be likely to hear at present in many GPs' surgeries. This doctor is willing to use unorthodox as well as conventional remedies. He knows their limitations as well as their strengths. He is also happy to swap patients from one to the other in an attempt to find the best way of tackling a particular problem. In short, he takes each approach on its merits. Is this how medicine could and perhaps should be practised in the future? I think so – though I'm far from certain that it actually will be in the next few years. Some of the difficulties and hurdles are pure prejudice; but others are real enough.

Before considering the future prospects, let me reiterate the core of the argument, and why an awareness of the placebo effect is central to it. Both doctors and complementary practitioners want the same thing: to eliminate disease at source or, failing that, to minimize its consequences; to 'please the patient', as I've described it. Orthodox practitioners set about the task using techniques chosen for their specific pharmacological or physiological actions. They are well aware of the existence of non-material influences over the body's own healing processes; they are aware, that is, of the placebo effect. But while their attempts to discount it when carrying out clinical research are reasonable and appropriate, the virtual neglect of this useful phenomenon by so many doctors in their routine practice is perverse. In this sense most doctors make little conscious effort to please their patients.

Unorthodox practitioners – some of whom have had little formal scientific training, and most of whom do not think about what they do in the terms of science – work in ways that, consciously or instinctively, tend to maximize the placebo action of their techniques. The rising popularity of this sort of medicine is one indication that these practitioners are indeed pleasing their patients. There is nothing pejorative in the claim that they are putting the placebo effect to good use – and this remains the case whether or not you believe that their therapies have specific actions over and above the placebo response.

If this *is* a fair description of the difference between doctors and their counterparts in complementary medicine, the conclusion must be that each group has something to learn from the other. And when rivals *can* bring themselves to accept such a thing, they've taken the first step towards co-operation. The second step is for both parties to accept their own weaknesses as well as the other's strengths. People with advanced kidney failure are foolish to put their trust exclusively in herbalism, acupuncture or homeopathy. None of these is likely to restore the lost kidney function; only dialysis (to take over the work of the kidney) or transplantation (to replace it) will save their lives. But someone whose low back pain has been treated unsuccessfully for years by conventional medicine is equally foolish to restrict him or herself to analgesics and hospital-approved physiotherapy when osteopathy, acupuncture or chiropractic might do the trick.

As I pointed out in the introduction to this book, a great deal of the illness that confronts GPs is of the chronic and degenerative type (rheumatoid arthritis, for example) in which treatment – if it works at all – is little more than a holding operation. If the doctor succeeds in eliminating pain, he's doing well; if he manages to slow the progress of the disease, he deserves medals. Most often, of course, pain is mitigated rather than eliminated; and the disease continues to progress. Another part of the GP's workload consists of dealing with patients with chronic anxiety, recurrent bouts of depression and other minor psychiatric disorders. Drugs may help, but it doesn't require a great deal of insight to appreciate that drug therapy is often given with the hope of papering over the cracks rather than with any conviction that the problem is being tackled at root.

In these and other circumstances, the 'body technician' role of the GP soon runs out of steam. And when feelings of general unhappiness or frustration or some other such state of mind are what brings the patient, *faute de mieux*, in search of medical help, the body technician role has no useful part to play. Complementary medicine, on the other hand, with its emphasis on the individuality of the patient and the importance of listening, and its disinclination to make hard and fast distinctions between mental and physical distress, may still have something to offer.

Many patients seem to sense that there is a place for more than one approach to disease and dis-ease. It is the doctors who need to be convinced.

Bridging the gap

An awareness of the placebo effect can serve as a valuable bridge between complementary and orthodox medicine. It is a powerful and persuasive demonstration that states of mind are an important determinant of physical health: powerful because of the sheer scale of the effect; and, as far as doctors are concerned, powerfully persuasive as a way of changing attitudes towards unorthodox medicine because the phenomenon is so utterly respectable! In polite company, where talk of herbalism, hypnotherapy, homeopathy and healing might raise eyebrows, the placebo effect can be discussed without fear of frightening the horses or calling into question anyone's scientific credentials. The concept should be equally attractive to complementary practitioners because it offers a sound theoretical underpinning for their style of medicine. To those who sneer that complementary techniques are *of their nature* unscientific, practitioners have a powerful rebuttal. They can point out – as they do – that there is nothing irrational or unscientific about trying to mobilize the body's own healing mechanisms; to this they can now add some expression of regret that orthodox medical science has yet to make as much progress in understanding these systems as complementary medical practitioners have already made in exploiting them!

Because a capacity to induce the placebo effect is the exclusive property of neither group, it should remind both of what they have in common. Insofar as any practitioner – orthodox or complementary – is exercising an influence on his or her patient that goes beyond the specific actions of the remedy, that practitioner is exploiting the placebo effect. To suggest that there are no distinctions to be made between orthodox and complementary practitioners would be absurd. But they do have enough in common to understand each other and – most important – to work together.

The right time

Change seldom occurs, and even less often takes root, unless circumstances have first prepared the ground. Two factors are currently smoothing the path towards a mutual acceptance of orthodox and complementary medicines. One is the rising public enthusiasm for the latter. The 1986 BMA report on alternative medicine speculated (as much in hope as expectation?) that interest in unorthodox techniques might be a 'passing fashion'. If it is indeed a fashion, it hasn't passed yet. Indeed, by almost every measure – opinion polls, numbers of practitioners and consultations, the variety of books on the topic being published and financial turnover – the growth of complementary medicine has not yet peaked.

The second factor that is serving, albeit quite incidentally, to pave the way for complementary medicine is a rising awareness within orthodox medicine of the importance of quality as well as quantity of life. Conventional medicine has always tended to judge its success by criteria such as the extension of life and the prevention of premature death because these outcomes are easy to define and to measure. Patients are either alive or they are not; it is a tidy distinction that leaves little room for dispute. Their obsession with death prevention has sometimes led doctors to do things that their patients have not sought. The dose of pneumonia ('old man's friend') that can quietly terminate a life that has already become burdensome is still, on occasion, fought off with antibiotics; terminal cancer may be resisted using treatments that do nothing other than add a few months to a life that has already become intolerable. That these things happen less often than they used to is largely because doctors *have* become more aware of the importance of quality of life.

Medicine being the scientific occupation it is, ingenious attempts are even now being made to quantify that term 'quality of life'. This endeavour has led to a new word: the 'QALY', an acronym derived from 'quality adjusted life year'. The thinking behind this is that one year of healthy life may be worth two or three or more years of life spent in a diseased or otherwise debilitated condition. The performance of medicine can then be judged not only in terms of the number of calendar years of life added by this or that procedure, but by the number of QALYs it offers. The obvious question is how you calculate the relationship between a calendar year and a QALY. Would you trade two years of life as a quadraplegic for one of healthy existence? Or would you think it appropriate to sacrifice three or four or even more years of such an existence for one healthy one?

The only way to find out is to ask people. Indeed, the QALY system is based on just such a survey. A group of people were asked to rate, on a scale from nought to 100, the extent to which a range of disabilities would reduce their quality of life. These scores provided the conversion factors for translating calendar years into QALYs in a range of distressing and disabling mental and physical conditions. (One interesting finding that emerged from this exercise was that certain conditions ended up with a negative score; in other words, the general view was that death would be preferable to life in these particular circumstances.) The QALY is a fairly primitive instrument, and still controversial; but it is already showing that quality of life is a concept tangible enough to be taken into account.

For the present, though, doctors continue to judge most of their performance on the basis of cure. If the patient has a tumour that neither drugs nor radiotherapy can eliminate, the doctor will probably feel he or she has laboured in vain. Premature death equals failure. The advent of hospices represented a belated realization of the need for the development of formal expertise in the care of the dying. But even now medicine has relatively little to offer those whose illnesses, while not terminal, disrupt and undermine their lives. Hence the value of an organization like the Blackthorn Trust.

The complementary therapist, by having less ambitious expectations about eliminating acute illness or saving life, may not feel that death is quite the personal failure it seems to many doctors. If the remainder of a patient's life is passed in a state of reasonable physical comfort and mental tranquillity, most complementary practitioners wouldn't feel they had failed their patients. The aromatherapist who makes regular visits to a hospital specializing in the care of people with AIDS feels no sense of guilt. At risk of alienating the many doctors for whom this isn't true, I will say that the importance of quality of life has more often been apparent to patients and to complementary practitioners than it has to the medical profession. Comparisons between the QALY scores for complementary as opposed to orthodox medicine would make fascinating reading.

Mutual recognition

In principle, the swiftest and simplest escape from the present hostility between conventional and unorthodox medicine would be for the medical establishment to declare its recognition that complementary medicine has something to offer, and to open a dialogue on matters such as training, registration and co-operation. This would be fine so far as it went. But if no other changes were to be made, the resulting position would be one in which the State, through the NHS, funded the vast majority of orthodox medicine, while all but a fraction of complementary medicine was still private. The complementary practitioners would argue that, if their therapies were to be regarded as acceptable, then they too should be eligible for employment within the NHS – either as salaried staff like hospital doctors, or as independent contractors like GPs. The Government would have a view on the matter, for reasons of cost if for no other. As a significant proportion of patients using complementary medicine are also using conventional medicine, the Government couldn't hope that the cost of new funds for the one would be wholly offset by a reduction in demand for the other. There probably would be some reduction – but it certainly wouldn't cover all the new expenditure.

A more radical change would be to have complementary therapists and doctors practising together. When most GPs practised single handed or in pairs, such co-operation might have been more difficult than it would be today. With larger partnerships, and with several practices sometimes sharing the same bigger and better endowed health centres, close collaboration with unorthodox practitioners becomes a more realistic possibility. This is not the place in which to discuss the particulars, financial and otherwise, of such relationships; some general points do need to be addressed, however.

There is, for example, the issue of who is in control. Some complementary practitioners whose educational standards are indisputably high – the European College of Chiropractic in Bournemouth, for example, now offers a degree course recognized by the Council for National Academic Awards – would be well-placed to seek acceptance by the NHS. But short of a dramatic change of heart by the medical profession, their role would almost certainly be subsidiary to that of the doctor. In other words, people with low back pain would go first to their GP, who would then decide whether to refer them to the hospital for conventional medicine or to, say, an NHS-funded chiropractor. In this respect, the chiropractors – in common with most other complementary practitioners – wish to remain as they are now: health care workers from whom the public can seek help without having first to be referred by a doctor. They argue that conventionally trained doctors aren't in a position to know which patients might benefit from complementary medicine, so to have GPs acting as the gatekeepers would be wasteful if not obstructive.

The doctors would argue with equal force that the British system – in which nearly all approaches to specialists of whatever kind are mediated by GPs – ensures that patients are directed towards people with the appropriate skills, and that giving the family doctor this pivotal position guarantees that there is always one person who has an overview of the health of any particular patient.

A more fundamental objection to the whole notion of trying to unify orthodox and alternative medicine might be that part of the appeal and indeed the success of the latter *is* that it lies outside the mainstream and is therefore in some way 'special'. Any such feeling among patients is likely to exert a powerful placebo effect – which would be correspondingly lost if all complementary therapists were to become just another group of health workers. Short of surrounding this branch of health care with artificial boundaries – more or less the very opposite of what is being advocated in this book – the risk is one that would just have to be run.

Doctors' dilemma

If complementary medicine *is* to be given a recognized status, there will be some doctors who find themselves in a predicament. What are they to do when confronted by a patient asking to be referred to a therapist offering an unorthodox treatment in which they themselves have no faith? If they believed the therapy to be actively harmful, they would have a duty to refuse. In practice this will seldom arise; few complementary therapies have adverse effects. More commonly, doctors will find themselves asked to refer their patients for treatments that they simply don't believe to have any value beyond that of a placebo.

This will be tricky for them to deal with, but not impossible. Knowing, as they will, about the power of the placebo effect they will be aware that some at least of those patients who receive the treatment will benefit from it, even if it doesn't have any specific beneficial effects on the body. They will also be aware that emphasizing their own scepticism too openly may undermine that placebo effect, and thus do their patients no service. In these circumstances it would surely be acceptable enough to use one of the standard formulae that tell no lies, but conceal what the doctor himself believes to be the truth. ('I've no experience myself of this therapy, but I've heard that some people find it helpful.')

The extent to which this is a problem will depend on the therapy in question. Doctors who believe that radionics is hocus pocus may well be exceedingly reluctant to see their patients pursuing it. But those same doctors might have no hesitation in referring patients to a practitioner offering traditional Chinese acupuncture. You don't have to accept the theory of Chinese medicine with its meridians and energy channels to believe that acupuncture has effects on the body. To take a somewhat extravagant parallel, you don't have to believe in God to feel a sense of reverence when entering a great cathedral. The fact that there is often room to debate the nature and causes of a phenomenon is not always to deny its existence.

Much the same is true of the work of the Blackthorn Trust described in the previous chapter. Rudolf Steiner, the philosopher whose writings inspired the formation of the Trust, believed that living things could not be explained in purely physical and chemical terms. In addition to our physical bodies he maintained that we have what he called 'etheric' bodies, which allow us to grow and to restore ourselves. He also wrote of an 'astral' body associated with thought, perception and self-awareness. It need hardly be said that none of this makes much sense to scientific orthodoxy. But, again, you don't have to accept Steiner's own view of the matter to appreciate that patients benefit from the art and music therapies offered by the Trust. All theory aside, a determination to treat people humanely would be enough to justify such activities.

Some doctors – through prejudice, or in response to a sincere but misconceived idea that if medicine is to retain its scientific purity it must reject all unorthodox forms of treatment – will go on refusing to countenance any acceptance of complementary techniques. What to say to such individuals? How best to breach the barrier and arouse at least some sympathy?

If orthodox medicine was able to deal with all the problems that patients bring to their doctors, a refusal to have any truck with the unconventional might be justified. But orthodox medicine is not omnipotent, and when doctors have tried their best and failed to deal with problems, be they purely medical or partly psychosocial, can they still justify refusing to grant complementary medicine the opportunity to at least try? Some doctors, even those who accept that many of their own patients have unfulfilled needs, do take this attitude. Pressed to account for the popularity of complementary medicine, and the benefits that many of its recipients claim for it, they will argue that they too could achieve as much if they had the one commodity that many of them obviously lack: time. If resources did become available, doctors who take this view would probably be inclined to set up a counselling service rather than seek a complementary therapist.

The only way of convincing such individuals that they might be wrong to fence themselves and their patients off from unorthodox medicine is to issue a challenge: as long as you have a single patient for whom the help you can offer is insufficient or inappropriate, how can you – in the best traditions of scientific medicine – deny the *possibility* that someone else using something different might succeed? Dressing an infected wound with a poultice of mouldy bread sounds pretty outlandish – until you recall that penicillin is produced by a mould. Doctors wondering whether to revise their attitude to the fringe should remember two things: first, many practices once considered unconventional are now orthodox; and second, you don't have to believe all the claims made by the more enthusiastic propagandists of this or that complementary technique to accept that there might be a jot of truth in it, and give it a try. It is not necessary to become totally credulous or to abandon science when putting the first exploratory toe in the waters of complementary medicine. Science demands that you retain your scepticism; but science also demands that you first investigate.

At risk of perpetrating a heresy, it could even be argued that there are some things that don't have to be scientifically validated. To the extent that a system of treatment makes specific promises to cure specific diseases, its claims do need to be tested. But if its aim is simply to increase the recipient's sense of well-being, the full panoply of science's experimental methodology need not be wielded. We do not organize elaborate experiments to find out if people prefer television to the cinema, enjoy white wine more than red, or get more pleasure from Jane Austen than Frederick Forsythe; we simply ask. Feeling good is a subjective judgement; so the most reliable judge of that condition is the individual him or herself.

This, perhaps, is the point at which medicine-as-science parts company with medicine-as-art. These last are weasel words, too often used to cloak sloppy thinking and disguise ill-thought-out intentions. But they do also have a legitimate use; medicine is about human beings trying to deal with one anothers' problems and, as in other human relationships, the quality of the interaction is not easily dissected, categorized, and quantified. It could be said that medicine-as-science is primarily concerned with ends, and medicine-as-art with means. It might be added that many of the differences between orthodox and non-orthodox medicine can be categorized in roughly the same way. The hospital doctor aims for swift solutions to defined problems; the complementary practitioner is just as concerned with the way in which those ends are pursued, believing that the ends themselves will anyway be attained only if the means are appropriate. Pursuing that same divide still further, orthodox medicine aims to treat disease, assuming that a state of well-being will replace it. Complementary medicine may make the pursuit of well-being an end in itself, with disease being elbowed out of existence *en route*. Indeed, some of the goals of complementary medicine bear little relation to those of conventional medicine. Despite the substantial overlap in the intentions of the two enterprises, it is not altogether surprising that they sometimes seem to be travelling on parallel but unconnected tracks.

The weakness of the pragmatic approach to any system of

health care ('If it works, use it') lies in the risk of casting aside all the cherished ideals of scientific medicine. I have pointed out that useful knowledge is seldom acquired without effort, and that to abandon the rigour of science – a rigour that has brought so many proven benefits – would be a tragic mistake. Hence the narrow (but understandable) response of those doctors who ask why scientific medicine should make *any* accommodation with the fringe, and say to their unorthodox counterparts, 'Come back and tell us about your techniques when you've made the effort to validate them. We'll take an interest – but only when you show us the evidence.'

The pragmatic approach is indeed saying that if this or that patient is happy with this or that treatment, and actually benefits by it, what else matters? As far as any individual whose treatment has been successful is concerned, this is fine. But in wider terms the medical scientists are right: such anti-intellectualism simply will not do. *Did* the treatment itself achieve something, or was it purely a placebo response? This issue matters because, much as the benefits of a placebo effect are to be welcomed, the greater benefits of a placebo effect *plus* a specific action against the disease in question are to be welcomed even more. If the treatment really *is* more than a placebo, could the specific effects it does have be improved upon by altering it in some way? Unless these questions are repeatedly addressed, any system of medicine fossilizes. For centuries, physicians uncritically accepted and passed on a whole series of misunderstandings about the body in health and disease because the custom of the times was to accept the writings of one man, the Roman physician Galen, as if they were holy writ. One of the glories of science is its inbuilt mechanism for challenging received wisdom, and refining it. This healthy attitude is less evident in complementary medicine where the tendency is still to accept what is taught rather than to question it.

Equally important as a reason for questioning unorthodox therapies is the need to guard against conscious fraud. The placebo effect offers the unscrupulous a tempting opportunity to devise bogus therapies. Anyone with a passing knowledge of the phenomenon, a plausible manner, and a little imagination should, without difficulty, be able to cobble together a reasonably convincing system of treatment. If it pleases the patients, a third of them will then experience benefits – quite sufficient for a flourishing practice.

A conditional *rapprochement*

It follows that any *rapprochement* between orthodox and complementary medicine should be conditional upon the latter agreeing to several important developments. One of these would have to be that complementary practitioners put more effort into validating the claims they make for their techniques. They should also strive to improve the effectiveness of their therapies using the kind of experimental assessment that is commonplace in orthodox science and medicine. In the case of a number of the major therapies, such as acupuncture, chiropractic and homeopathy, this would be pushing at an open door. There would also have to be a systematic attempt to agree on professional standards and educational requirements within each branch of complementary medicine. Some recognized form of statutory registration would be the ideal but, given that many practitioners who belong to only one of the various professional bodies in the field may use several different techniques, this would not be without problems. Someone who is primarily an acupuncturist may use homeopathy and vice versa. The difficulties created by inter-professional rivalries and jealousies should never be underestimated.

There are, of course, one or two quid pro quos here. Complementary practitioners will wish orthodox physicians to recall that not all *their* therapies have been subject to the kind of critical assessment that they themselves advocate. And given the resources and expertise available to orthodox medicine, complementary practitioners would be entitled to seek assistance in organizing the experimental validation that I have argued is essential. Doctors may also wish to start taking the implications of the placebo effect more seriously in their day-to-day work. Insofar as the placebo effect grows out of the patients' faith in their doctors and in the treatment they are receiving, anything that doctors can do to boost that faith should stimulate the healing process. Doctors must, however reluctantly, learn to think of themselves once more as healers, and behave accordingly. The demands of this role are not necessarily onerous: to expect politeness, sympathy, and respect for patients is hardly to place an unreasonable burden on the profession. More difficult to fulfil are the patients' needs to take things at their own pace; to believe that the doctor is prepared to listen to what they have to say, and to take it seriously. Some will, of course, never be satisfied; but more could be.

If and when various unorthodox techniques are demonstrated to everyone's satisfaction as efficacious, some doctors – those whose interest in medicine is primarily in what I've called 'body technology' – will still be happy to leave their use to non-medically trained individuals. But others will surely argue that it should be the exclusive responsibility of the medical profession to adopt them. Aside from any lack of inclination to get involved, there are several arguments for not putting most complementary techniques in the hands of most doctors. Their training does not currently (and forseeably) suit them to perform this kind of work. Whether public or private it is impossible to imagine circumstances in which more than a handful of doctors could routinely offer the thirty or forty minutes that most complementary practitioners devote to each patient. And for doctors regularly to spend, say, half an hour massaging someone's body with aromatic oils would be an absurd waste of a long, expensive and highly technical training.

Something for everyone

If some kind of mutual acceptance can be reached there are potential gains for patients and for practitioners, both orthodox and complementary. Patients won't find themselves having to negotiate with two opposed systems. They would no longer be fearful of a real or imagined reprimand if the doctor found out that they were also receiving unorthodox treatment. Recognition would also strengthen the hand of those within complementary medicine who are disturbed by the current lack of registration and control of standards. Charlatans would find it harder to thrive. It would also help to bring about the improvement of the techniques themselves, many of which have yet to be subject to proper scrutiny. And in so far as the State might choose to make at least some therapies available under the NHS, patients would have a broader choice.

Complementary practitioners, too, would benefit in respect of this last point. Their training might become eligible for State funding and they would no longer be on the receiving end of the periodic sniping they now have to endure from the doctors. Orthodox physicians would be relieved of some of the burden of the many patients for whom they can do little: people with chronic physical ailments for which there is no satisfactory remedy; people with minor psychiatric disturbances; people who are simply unhappy or unable to cope. All these would have something to gain from freer and easier access to complementary medicine.

These changes would not be without discomfort or even pain on both sides. Those doctors who are comfortable with the role of scientist-cum-body technician will not welcome any greater emphasis on the human element in what they do. The burden of change to be borne by complementary practitioners, and in particular the development of a more self-critical view of their methods and ideas, will probably prove even more demanding. It is difficult to believe that *all* their weird and wonderful techniques will turn out to have quite as many specific benefits as they now claim.

To choose an example at random and without prejudice, it might one day be shown that aromatherapists have overinterpreted the differences between the effects of using one oil as against another. In claiming that geranium is particularly useful for viral infections and urinary disorders, fennel for digestive problems and kidney stones, and rosemary for poor memory, mental fatigue and rheumatism, aromatherapists may be exaggerating the importance of the difference between one oil and another. Does this mean that aromatherapy is useless? Certainly not. At the very least, different patients will have preferences for different oils; and the greater part of what the aromatherapist does, the application of the oil as part of a system of massage, indisputably pleases many people in pain, discomfort or distress. I am not suggesting that aromatherapy *will* have to modify its claims; I have no idea. What I am suggesting is that even if it did have to, it could still play a role. Much the same would be true of many other complementary techniques.

Patients, too, should play more than a passive role in forging these new attitudes. Faith in the practitioner and the therapies on offer is valuable; but a blind, credulous, unquestioning faith is less helpful than one based on understanding. Let patients therefore ask their doctors and their complementary practitioners to explain what is being recommended and why.

The goal, in short, must be a new outlook in health care: one in which techniques are judged on their merit, not on preconceived notions of what medicine should be about. The aim must be to develop a blend of health care that is no less scientific than today's orthodox medicine, and no less caring than complementary medicine, but more effective than either. Then will patients be truly 'pleased'.

References

This list is not exhaustive; it includes only the key references.

1 Pink Pills and Friendly Physicians

Balint, M., 'The doctor, his patient, and the illness', *Lancet* (1955), 1, pp. 283–688.

Huskisson, E. C., 'Simple analgesics for arthritis', *British Medical Journal* (1974), 4, pp. 196–200.

Memmeshiemer, A. M., et al., 'Untersuchungen uber die suggestive behandlung der warzen', *Dermatologische Zeitschrift* (1931), 62, pp. 63–8.

2 A Tiresome Distraction

Beecher, H. K., 'The powerful placebo', *Journal of the American Medical Association* (1955), 159, pp. 1602–6.

— 'Surgery as placebo: a quantitative study of bias', *Journal of the American Medical Association* (1961), 176, pp. 1102–7.

Benson, H., and McCallie, D. P., 'Angina pectoris and the placebo effect', *New England Journal of Medicine* (1979), 300, pp. 1424–9.

Blackwell, B., et al., 'Demonstration to medical students of placebo responses and non-drug factors', *Lancet* (1972), 1, pp. 1279–82.

Branthwaite, A., and Cooper, P., 'Analgesic effects of branding in treatment of headaches', *British Medical Journal* (1981), 282, pp. 1576–8.

Cobb, L. A., et al., 'An evaluation of internal mammary artery ligation by a double-blind technique', *New England Journal of Medicine* (1959), 260, pp. 1115–8.

Dimond, E. G., 'Comparison of internal mammary artery ligation and sham operation for angina pectoris', *American Journal of Cardiology* (1960), 5, pp. 483–6.

Ellis, L. G., et al., 'Long-term management of patients with coronary artery disease', *Circulation* (1958), 17, pp. 945–52.

Feldman, P., 'The personal element in psychiatric research', *American Journal of Psychiatry* (1956), 113, pp. 52–4.

Huskisson, E. C., 'Simple analgesics for arthritis', *British Medical Journal* (1974), 4, pp. 196–200.

Mitchell, J. R., 'Bilateral internal mammary artery ligation for angina pectoris: preliminary clinical considerations', *Annals of Surgery* (1960), 152, pp. 325–9.

Schapira, K., et al., 'Study of the effect of tablet colour on the treatment of anxiety', *British Medical Journal* (1970), 2, pp. 446–9.

Shapiro, A. K., 'A contribution to the history of the placebo effect', *Behavioural Science* (1960), 5, pp. 109–35.

Vinar, O., 'Dependence on a placebo: a case report', *British Journal of Psychiatry* (1969), 115, pp. 1189–90.

3 The Healing Mind

Arnetz, B. B., et al., 'Immune function in unemployed women', *Psychosomatic Medicine* (1987), 49, pp. 3–12.

Balint, M., 'The doctor, his patient, and the illness', *Lancet* (1955), 1, pp. 283–688.

Bartrop, R. W., et al., 'Depressed lymphocyte function after bereavement', *Lancet* (1977), 1, pp. 834–6.

Greer, S., and Moris, T., 'Psychological attributes of women who develop breast cancer', *Journal of Psychosomatic Research* (1975), 19, pp. 147–53.

Gryll, S., and Katahn, K., 'Situational factors contributing to the placebo effect', *Psychopharmacology* (1978), 57, pp. 253–61.

Haynes, R. B., et al., 'Increased absenteeism from work after detection and labelling of hypertensive patients', *New England Journal of Medicine*, 229, pp. 741–4.

Irwin, M., 'Depression and immune function', *Stress Medicine* (1988), 4, pp. 95–103.

Jemmott, J. B., et al., 'Academic stress, power motivation, and decrease in secretion rate of salivary secretory immunoglobulin A', *Lancet* (1983), 1, pp. 1400–2.

Kasl, S. V., et al., 'Psychosocial risk factors in the development of infectious mononucleosis', *Psychosomatic Medicine* (1979), 41, pp. 445–65.

Kiecolt-Glaser, J. K., et al., 'Urinary cortisol levels, cellular immunocompetency, and loneliness in psychiatric patients', *Psychosomatic Medicine* (1984), 49, pp. 15–22.

— 'Marital quality, marital disruption, and immune function', *Psychosomatic Medicine* (1987), 49, pp. 23–32.

Levine, J. D., et al., 'The mechanism of placebo analgesia', *Lancet* (1978), 2, pp. 654–7.

Spiegel, D., et al., 'Effect of psychosocial treatment on survival of patients with metastatic breast cancer', *Lancet* (1989), 2, pp. 888–91.

Ulrich, R., 'View through a window may influence recovery from surgery', *Science* (1984), 224, pp. 420–1.

4 Into the Consulting Rooms

Mendel, D., *Proper Doctoring*, Springer-Verlag, Vienna, 1984.

5 A Crooked Path

Porter, R. (ed.), *Man Masters Nature*, BBC, London, 1987.
Rhodes, P., *An Outline History of Medicine*, Butterworths, Oxford, 1985.
Ronan, C., *The Cambridge Illustrated History of the World's Science*, CUP, Cambridge, 1983.
Williams, G., *The Age of Miracles*, Constable, London, 1981.

6 A Series of Rebellions

Bagenal, F. S., et al., 'Survival of patients with breast cancer attending Bristol Cancer Help Centre', *Lancet* (1990), 336, pp. 606–10.

Davenas, E., et al., 'Human basophil degranulation triggered by very dilute anti-serum against IgE', *Nature* (1988), 333, pp. 816–8.

Gibson, S. L. M., et al., 'Homeopathic therapy in rheumatoid arthritis: evaluation by double-blind clinical therapeutic trial', *British Journal of Clinical Pharmacology* (1980), 9, p. 453.

Inglis, B., *Natural Medicine*, Collins, London, 1979.

Meade, T. W., et al., 'Low back pain of mechanical origin: randomised comparison of chiropractic and hospital outpatient treatment', *British Medical Journal* (1990), 300, pp. 1431–7.

Porter, R., *Health for Sale*, Manchester University Press, Manchester, 1989.

Steel, K., et al., 'Iatrogenic illness on a general medical service at a university hospital', *New England Journal of Medicine* (1981), 304, pp. 638–42.

Tobias, J., and Baum, M., 'Bristol Cancer Help Centre' (letter), *Lancet* (1990), 336, p. 1323.

7 Who Are the Healers Now?

BMA Board of Science, *Working party on alternative therapy*, British Medical Association, 1986.

Meade, T. W., et al., 'Low back pain of mechanical origin: randomised comparison of chiropractic and hospital outpatient treatment', *British Medical Journal* (1990), 300, pp. 1431–7.

Reilly, D. T., 'Young doctors' views on alternative medicine', *British Medical Journal* (1983), 287, pp. 337–9.

Sacks, O., *Awakenings*, Picador, London, 1990.

Wharton, R., and Lewith, G., 'Complementary medicine and the GP', *British Medical Journal* (1986), 292, pp. 1498–1500.

8 Harnessing the Placebo Effect

Bok, S., 'The ethics of giving placebos', *Scientific American* (1974), 231 (5), pp. 17–23.

Campbell, A., *The two faces of homeopathy*, Jill Norman, London, 1984.

Christensen et al., 'Electroacupuncture and postoperative pain', *British Journal of Anaesthesia* (1989), 62, pp. 258–62.

Coan et al., 'The acupuncture treatment of low back pain: a randomised controlled study', *American Journal of Chinese Medicine* (1980), 8, pp. 181–9.

Goodwin, J. S., et al., 'Knowledge and use of placebos by house officers and nurses', *Annals of Internal Medicine* (1979), 197, pp. 106–10.

Kleijnen, J., et al., 'Clinical trials of homeopathy', *British Medical Journal* (1991), 302, pp. 316–23.

Reilly, D., et al., 'Is homeopathy a placebo response? Controlled trial of homeopathic potency, with pollen in hay fever as model', *Lancet* (1986), 2, pp. 881–6.

Shapiro, A. K., 'A contribution to the history of the placebo effect', *Behavioural Science* (1960), 5, pp. 109–35.

9 Mainstream Meets the Fringe

Budd, C., et al., 'A model of co-operation between complementary and allopathic medicine in a primary care setting', *British Journal of General Practice* (1990), 40, pp. 376–8.

General

Ashley, J., *Anatomy of a Hospital*, OUP, Oxford, 1987.
Dixon, B., *What is Science For?*, Collins, London, 1973.
Fulder, S., *The Handbook of Complementary Medicine*, OUP, Oxford, 1988.
Helman, C., *Culture, Health and Illness*, John Wright, Bristol, 1985.
Illich, I., *Limits to Medicine*, Marion Boyars, London, 1976.
Inglis, B. and West, R., *The Alternative Health Guide*, Michael Joseph, London, 1983.
Ornstein, R. and Sobel, D., *The Healing Brain*, Macmillan, London, 1988.
Pietroni, P., *The Greening of Medicine*, Gollancz, London, 1988.
Totman, R., *Social Causes of Illness*, Souvenir Press, London, 1979.
— *Mind, Stress and Health*, Souvenir Press, London, 1990.

Index

Aberdeen, University of, 34
Abrams, Albert, 80
abstinence syndrome, 36
acupuncture: BMA report, 112; equipment, 103; foot injury, 56; GP attitudes, 115, 140, 141, 157; pain control, 36, 104, 134–5; status, 81, 86, 161; uses, 150
adrenalin, 45, 98
adrenocorticotrophic hormone (ACTH), 44
AIDS, 26, 69, 107, 145–7, 154
'alternative medicine', 81
Amerindians, 60
anaesthesia (anaesthetic), 21, 67
analgesia (analgesics), 14–15, 36–7; *see also* pain control
angina, 3–5, 11–12, 16, 22, 98–9
Anglo-European College of Chiropractic, Bournemouth, 138, 155
antibiotics, 119, 121
Anti-Quackery Society, 77
Arabic medicine, 63
Aristotle, 23, 62
aromatherapy, 103, 135, 145–7, 154, 163–4
Aromatherapy in Care, 145
art therapy, 142–3, 144, 157
arthritis: homeopathy studies, 86, 131, 134; Hoxton Health Group, 145; number of sufferers xi; placebo studies, 14–15, 131; treatment, 70, 142, 150
aspirin, 14–15, 83, 131
association, 24
asthma, 69, 135
Atlanta, Georgia, 24
Auden, W. H., 38, 40
Australian Aborigines, 60
Austria, 79
Ayurvedic medicine, 71

Babylonian medicine, 61
back pain, 87, 131, 134, 150, 155
bacterial disease, 66, 69
Balint, Michael, x–xi, 18, 124
'basophil degranulation test', 87–8
Baum, Michael, 90
Beecher, Henry, 16, 22
Benson, Herbert, 11–12
Benveniste, Jacques, 87–8
bereavement, 38, 42, 43; counselling, 139
beta-blockers, 98
bitters, 121
'black box' investigation, 80–1
Blackthorn Trust, 141–4, 154, 157
blood pressure, 39, 133
Bok, Sissela, 122
Boston, Mass., 43
Boyle, Robert, 8, 64
brain, 31–2

INDEX

Branthwaite, A., 15
breast cancer, 40–2, 89–90
Bristol Cancer Help Centre (BCHC), 89–90
British College of Health, 78
British Journal of Psychiatry, 17
British Medical Association (BMA), 111–15, 128, 152
British Medical Journal, 38
bronchitis xi

California, University of, 36
Camden New Journal, 82
Campbell, Anthony, 132
cancer: Bristol Cancer Help Centre, 89–90; fear of, 53; mind and, 38, 40–2; radiotherapy, 96, 110; research, 70; treatments, 110, 152
caring for a relative, 45
case histories, 25–6
causation, 24
Center for Disease Control, Atlanta, 25
Centre for the Study of Alternative Therapies, 115
Charles, Prince of Wales, 111
Charles II, King, 8
chemical pollution, 83
chemicals, agricultural, 84
chemotherapy, 135
childbirth, 66, 101–2
Chinese medicine, 63, 157
chiropractic (chiropractors): low back pain trial, 86–7, 131, 134; origins, 79–80; status, 161; training, 155; use of technology, 103; uses, 150
chlorpromazine, 19, 125
Christianity, influence on medicine, 63, 71
Cincinnati University College of Medicine, 13
class influences, 144–5
Cobb, L. A., 4
cold fusion, 130
colour of tablets, 12–15

colour therapy, 115
complementary medicine, 51, 81–3, 103–7, 127–8, 151
contact, physical, 106
control groups, 120
Cooper, P., 15
Copernicus, 63
cortisol, 43–4
Council for Complementary and Alternative Medicine (CCAM), 110
Crick, Francis, 68
Crimean War, 67
Crockett, 4

Darwin, Charles, 65
Delaware, University of, 40
Denmark, 134
dental anaesthetic, 21
depression (depressives), 40, 43, 100
Descartes, René, 64
diagnosis, 105
diamorphine, 32
digitalis, 8
Dimond, E. G., 4
dissection, 71
divorce, 45; *see also* marriage
DNA, 68
doctors: as body technicians, 99–101, 139, 150, 162; as placebos, 18–22, 47, 124–6; attitudes to complementary medicine, 79, 115, 140–1, 157
'double-blind controlled trial', 28–9, 118, 130
dropsy, 8
drug: bills, 85, 140; therapy, 97–9, 110, 125, 150
duodenal ulcers, 22

Egyptian medicine, ancient, 7, 61
emotional disorders, xi
endorphins, 35–7
endoscope, 97
'energy flows', 105, 129–30
enkephalin, 34

INDEX

Epstein-Barr (EB) virus, 38–9
examination preparation, 43, 45

faith healing, 115
Feldman, Paul, 19
fibre-optics, 69
fibrositis, 86
Fields, Howard, 36–7
'fight or flight' response, 45
Fleischmann, Martin, 130
folk medicine, 74–5
food additives, 84
foxglove, 8
Franco, Francisco, 85
'fringe medicine', 81

Galen, 18, 63, 72, 160
Galileo, 64, 108–9
gallstones operation, 40, 69
General Medical Council, 68, 79, 114–15
genetic engineering, 68–9, 84
gentian mixture, 121
germ theory of disease, 65–7
glandular fever, 38–9
Glasgow study, 131
glyceryl trinitrate, 3
Gordon, Newton, 36–7
GPs, *see* doctors
Greek medicine, ancient, 7, 61–3, 71
green ideas, 83
Greer, Stephen, 40–1
Gryll, Steven, 21

Hahnemann, Samuel, 79
Harvard Medical School, Mass., 16
Harvey, William, 64
Hawthorne effect, 21, 91
hay fever, 86
headaches, 15
healers, 95, 108–9, 136–7
heart disease, 70
herbalism (herbalists): case study, 57–8; 'healer' role, 95; history, 74, 81; NHS relationship, 81, 140; uses, 150
herbs, 61, 107–8
hernia, hiatus, 57
heroin, 32, 34
Hippocrates, 25
Hippocratic Oath, 61–2
holistic principle, 104
homeopathy: arthritis study, 131, 134; GP attitudes, 79, 115, 140–1; origins, 79; status, 161; trials, 86, 134; use of technology, 103
Horder, Lord, 80
hormones, 33–4, 43–4, 45, 98
Hoxton Health Group, 144–5
Hughes, John, 34
humours, four, 62
Hunter, John, 65
Huskisson, Eric, 14
hydrotherapy, 56
Hygeian Journal, 78
hypertension, 39
hypnosis, 78, 115; self-, 41

iatrogenic illness, 85
iatroplacebogenesis, 20
Illich, Ivan, 85
immune defence system, 42–3
Industrial Revolution, 65
Inglis, Brian, 81
injections, 119
'inner states', 105
insulin, 33
intensive care, 96
internal mammary artery ligation, 3–5, 11, 22
International Federation of Aromatherapists, 135, 145

Jenner, Edward, 65

Katahn, Martin, 21
Keele, University of, 15
khellin, 11
kidney: failure, 150; stones, 97
King's Evil, the, 8

173

INDEX

Kittle, 4
knee problems, 51–2
Koch, Robert, 66
Kosterlitz, Hans, 34

Laennec, René Théophile Hyacinthe, 67
Lancet, x, 18, 77, 90
Largactil, 125
lasers, 96
L-dopa, 100–1
Leicester University Medical School, 126
Levine, Jon, 36–7
Lewith, George, 115–16
Lister, Joseph, 66–7
lymphocytes, 42

McCallie, David, 11–12
McGavin, David, 141–3
McMaster University, Canada, 39
macrophages, 42
malaria, 79
manipulation, 57, 79–80, 115
marriage: breakdown, 43, 45; guidance, 139
Marx, Karl, 65
Marylebone Health Centre, London, 140–1
maternal separation, 42
Medical Act (1858), 68
Medical Research Council, 86–7, 131
medicine, cost of, 85, 140
Mendel, David, 54
Mendel, Gregor, 68
Mesmer, Franz, 78
methadone, 32
methyl xanthines, 11
Middle Ages, 63
Minnesota Multiphasic Personality Inventory (MMPI), 40
monkeys, maternal separation, 42
Morison, James, 77–8
morphine, 32, 34
Mortality and Morbidity Weekly, 25
Murray, Geoffrey, 81

music therapy, 142–4, 157

naloxone, 34, 36–7
National Health Service (NHS): complementary therapy, 91, 140–1, 145–7, 154–5, 163; herbalists, 81; homeopathy, 79; 'limited list' of non-prescription medicines, viii, 121
'natural' medicine, 82–3
Nature, 88
naturopaths, 95
nerves, electrical stimulation, 36
neurotransmitters, 44
New Mexico, University of, 123
New York University College of Medicine, 117–18
Newcastle tablet colour study, 12–13
Newton, Isaac, 64
Newtonian physics, 91
Nightingale, Florence, 67
nitrous oxide, 67
nocebo effects, 16–18
nuclear energy, 83–4

obstetrics, 66, 101–2
opiate receptors, 33–4
opiates, 32–5
opium, 32
orthodox medicine: case studies, 51–5; definition, 62, 74; fringe split, 78; science and, 62, 71–2; *see also* doctors, surgery
osteopathy, 79–80, 140–1, 150
oxazepam, 12–13

pain: control, 16, 35–7, 41, *see also* analgesia; post-operative, 16, 123, 134–5
Palmer, D. D., 80
papaver somniferum, 32
Paracelsus, 9, 63
paracetamol, 14
Parkinson's disease, 142
participation in treatment, 106
Pasteur, Louis, 66

INDEX

Patel, Chandra, 133
Paul of Aegina, 7
penicillin, 129, 158
Pert, Candace, 33–4
pethidine, 32, 34
pet ownership, 46–7
pharmacology, 69
phenothiazines, 125
pill colour, 12–15
placebo effect, xii–xiii; attitudes to, 117–18, 127–30; definitions, 5–7; doctor as placebo, 18–22, 124–6; harnessing, 117–38, 160; history, 7–10; mechanism, 30–47; medical research, 27–9; tablet colour, 12–15; universal influence, 10–12
Pliny, 7
pneumonia, xi, 25, 152
Pomponazzi, Pierre, 9
Pons, Stanley, 130
poppy, opium, 32
Porter, Roy, 76, 77
post-operative pain, 16, 123, 134–5
Prague Psychiatric Research Institute, 17
pregnancy, 135
professionalism (doctors), 67–8
proof, 129–31
psychiatric patients, 43, 125, 142, 163
puerperal fever, 66

QALY (quality adjusted life year), 153–4
quacks, 74, 75, 76–8, 127–8
quality of life, 152–4
quantum theory, 91
Quimby, Dr, 10
quinine, 79

radioactivity, 83
radionics, 80–1, 112, 136, 157
radiotherapy, 96, 110
reflexologists, 95
Reilly, David Taylor, 115

relaxation, 133–4, 140
Renaissance, 63–4, 71, 74
Rivers, William, 10
Roman Empire, 63
Röntgen, Wilhelm Konrad von, 67
Royal Colleges, 67–8
Royal London Homeopathic Hospital, 132

Sacks, Oliver, 100–1
St Bartholomew's Hospital, London, 14
St Thomas's Hospital, London, 54, 67
Sargent, William, 125–6
schizophrenia, 17, 19, 21, 69, 125
science: flight from, 83–5; medicine and, 71–2
Scientific American, 122
scrofula, 8
Scutari, 67
seasickness, 16
self-hypnosis, 41
Semmelweiss, Ignaz Philipp, 66
Shapiro, Arthur, 5–6, 7, 10, 20, 117–18
skin disorders, xi
Smith, Sister Justa, 137
snake oil, 128
Snyder, Solomon, 33–4
Spiegal, David, 41
Stahl, Georg Ernst, 74
Stanford University, California, 41
steel worker study, 39
Steiner, Rudolf, 142, 157
stethoscope, 67
Still, Andrew, 80
strained ligaments, 56
stress, 38–9; glandular fever, 39; Hoxton Health Centre, 145; management, 133–4; mechanisms, 43–4; placebo effect, 46–7; trench mouth, 38; ubiquitous, 44–6
surgery: angina, 3–5, 11–12; complementary medicine's

175

INDEX

attitude to, 110; history, 61–5, 67, 97; technology, 97
Sydenham, London, 141

tablet colour, 12–15
Tavistock Clinic, London, 18
testicle lumps, 52–3
thalidomide, 81, 85
Third World, 70, 119
Tobias, Jeffrey, 90
Todd report, 126
tonics, 121
tooth extraction, 36–7
toothache, 7–8, 19
training, medical, 126–7, 154–5, 163
tranquillizers, 12–13, 57, 125
trench mouth, 38
trials, 27–9
Trudeau, Edward, 9
tuberculosis (TB), 8, 9–10, 66

ulcers, duodenal, 22
Ulrich, Roger, 40
ultrasound, 96–7
unemployment, 43
United States, 70, 80, 85, 134

upper respiratory tract disorders, xi
urban living, 45

Vegetable Universal pills, 77
Vinar, Oldrich, 17
viruses, 69, 121
vitalist approach, 73–5, 80–1
Vitamin E, 11
vivisection, 84

Wakeley, Thomas, 77–8
warts, viii
Wates Foundation, 141
Watson, James, 68
West Point Military Academy, 38–9
Wharton, Richard, 115–16
widowers and widows, 38
windows, view from, 40
'wise women', 74
witchcraft, 74
Withering, William, 8
Wolf, Stewart, 6

xanthines, 11
X-rays, 67, 96, 103

Yale University, 38